T0073676

Graphic Public Health

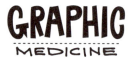

GRAPHIC MEDICINE

Susan Merrill Squier and Ian Williams, General Editors

Editorial Collective

MK Czerwiec (GraphicMedicine.org)
Michael J. Green (Penn State College of Medicine)
Kimberly R. Myers (Penn State College of Medicine)
Scott T. Smith (Penn State University)

Books in the Graphic Medicine series are inspired by a growing awareness of the value of comics as an important resource for communicating about a range of issues broadly termed "medical." For healthcare practitioners, patients, families, and caregivers dealing with illness and disability, graphic narrative enlightens complicated or difficult experience. For scholars in literary, cultural, and comics studies, the genre articulates a complex and powerful analysis of illness, medicine, and disability and a rethinking of the boundaries of "health." The series includes original comics from artists and non-artists alike, such as self-reflective "graphic pathographies" or comics used in medical training and education, as well as monographic studies and edited collections from scholars, practitioners, and medical educators.

Other titles in the series:

MK Czerwiec, Ian Williams, Susan Merrill Squier, Michael J. Green, Kimberly R. Myers, and Scott T. Smith, *Graphic Medicine Manifesto*

Ian Williams, *The Bad Doctor: The Troubled Life and Times of Dr. Iwan James*

Peter Dunlap-Shohl, *My Degeneration: A Journey Through Parkinson's*

Aneurin Wright, *Things to Do in a Retirement Home Trailer Park: . . . When You're 29 and Unemployed*

Dana Walrath, *Aliceheimers: Alzheimer's Through the Looking Glass*

Lorenzo Servitje and Sherryl Vint, eds., *The Walking Med: Zombies and the Medical Image*

Henny Beaumont, *Hole in the Heart: Bringing Up Beth*

MK Czerwiec, *Taking Turns: Stories from HIV/AIDS Care Unit 371*

Paula Knight, *The Facts of Life*

Gareth Brookes, *A Thousand Coloured Castles*

Jenell Johnson, ed., *Graphic Reproduction: A Comics Anthology*

Olivier Kugler, *Escaping Wars and Waves: Encounters with Syrian Refugees*

Judith Margolis, *Life Support: Invitation to Prayer*

Ian Williams, *The Lady Doctor*

Sarah Lightman, *The Book of Sarah*

Benjamin Dix and Lindsay Pollock, *Vanni: A Family's Struggle through the Sri Lankan Conflict*

Ephameron, *Us Two Together*

Scott T. Smith and José Alaniz, eds., *Uncanny Bodies: Superhero Comics and Disability*

MK Czerwiec, ed., *Menopause: A Comic Treatment*

Susan Merrill Squier and Irmela Marei Krüger-Fürhoff, eds., *PathoGraphics: Narrative, Aesthetics, Contention, Community*

Swann Meralli and Deloupy, *Algériennes: The Forgotten Women of the Algerian Revolution*

Aurélien Ducoudray and Jeff Pourquié, *The Third Population*

Abby Hershler, Lesley Hughes, Patricia Nguyen, and Shelley Wall, eds., *Looking at Trauma: A Tool Kit for Clinicians*

Kimberly R. Myers, Molly L. Osborne, Charlotte A. Wu, and Zoe Schein, *Clinical Ethics: A Graphic Medicine Casebook*

GRAPHIC PUBLIC HEALTH

A COMICS ANTHOLOGY AND ROAD MAP

MEREDITH LI-VOLLMER

The Pennsylvania State University Press | University Park, Pennsylvania

Library of Congress Cataloging-in-Publication Data

Names: Li-Vollmer, Meredith, author.
Title: Graphic public health : a comics anthology and road map / Meredith Li-Vollmer.
Other titles: Graphic medicine
Description: University Park, Pennsylvania : The Pennsylvania State University Press, [2022] | Series: Graphic medicine | Includes bibliographical references.
Summary: "Demonstrates how comics can address topics such as disease outbreaks, opioid addiction prevention, healthcare reform, and climate change while eliciting empathy, clarifying complexity, and broadening perspectives"—Provided by publisher.
Identifiers: LCCN 2021061032 | ISBN 9780271093253 (paperback : alk. paper)
Subjects: MESH: Health Education | Graphic Novels as Topic | Graphic Novel
Classification: LCC RA440.6 | NLM WA 17 | DDC 362.1071—dc23/eng/20220113
LC record available at https://lccn.loc.gov/2021061032

Printed in the United States of America
Published by The Pennsylvania State University Press, University Park, PA 16802–1003

The Pennsylvania State University Press is a member of the Association of University Presses.

It is the policy of The Pennsylvania State University Press to use acid-free paper. Publications on uncoated stock satisfy the minimum requirements of American National Standard for Information Sciences—Permanence of Paper for Printed Library Material, ANSI Z39.48–1992.

To my parents, scientists

who encouraged their

children to be creative

Contents

Acknowledgments

Thank you to all of the artists who have collaborated with me over the years and who generously gave permission to share their work in this anthology. To my friends in Comics Fever, thank you for introducing me to the thriving Seattle independent comics community and making me feel so welcome. I owe particular gratitude to Kelly Froh and David Lasky for mentoring me in the comics medium and encouraging me to make comics on my own.

Thank you to my incredible colleagues at Public Health—Seattle & King County and my Communications Team family, past and present. You inspire me every day, and I am so grateful to work with such talented and passionate people. James Apa and Carina Elsenboss, thank you for your early support of my experiments with comics (even if you weren't quite sure what I was up to initially) and for championing graphic public health in the department and to funders. I couldn't have done this work without you backing me. Thanks to Nicole Sadow-Hasenberg for reading very early drafts of my manuscript and Haley Raspet for coming to my rescue with formatting image files.

Several graduate students from the University of Washington have helped with the development and formative testing of my comics projects over the years. Thanks to all who helped, most especially Matthew French and Nikki Eller.

Stacy Pigg, thank you for your generosity in providing thoughtful feedback that helped me listen more closely to my own voice. My gratitude also to Susan Merrill Squier and Kendra Boileau for encouraging me to write this book.

And to my husband Alex, my daughter Audrey, my parents Judy and Hiram, and my brother Eric: thank you for allowing me to occasionally depict you in my comics for the greater public health good or just for my own amusement, and for your unwavering support that has held me up through two pandemics as well as all the rhythms of our lives together.

Introduction

I wrote my first comic book, *No Ordinary Flu*, in 2008 for the health department in Seattle. It was about preparing for an influenza pandemic. As I write this introduction in 2021, it's been more than a year since a real pandemic began in the United States, with the first reported case of novel coronavirus entering through the airport in the Seattle area. It's been surreal to see scenes from *No Ordinary Flu* unfold in real life: schools closed, empty sports arenas, lonely cubicles in office spaces.

My intent in developing *No Ordinary Flu* had been to help people visualize and mentally rehearse a possible public health crisis that was then hard for most people to fathom. At the time that I wrote and storyboarded this comic, few people were aware that a pandemic of the magnitude of the 1918 flu—or COVID-19—could even happen. Working with artist David Lasky, we used comics to show the scale of disruption and make the threat of a pandemic more tangible. Given the toll that COVID-19 has had on every aspect of our well-being, there's little gratification in seeing how closely the scenes we created in *No Ordinary Flu* mirror the reality of a global pandemic in 2020. But it does demonstrate the power of comics to accurately convey public health issues that are complex and enormously consequential.

More than a decade after *No Ordinary Flu*, and in the midst of a public health crisis more far reaching than I had even imagined, a sea change may be on the horizon in the public's relationship with public health issues. Jargon like "personal protective equipment," "social distancing," and "contact tracing" has entered the mainstream, and public health officials like Dr. Anthony Fauci have become celebrities. While the urgency of public health funding and support have finally been in the spotlight, the pandemic has also made visible long-standing health disparities. Support for public health has not been universal, with politicians and interest groups weaponizing public health measures to wedge further divisions between people.

Our experience during COVID-19 has also shown that everyone has a personal story to tell about public health. Our social media feeds, dinner conversations, and Zoom calls are filled with anecdotes about what happened when schools and work went remote, how it felt to get a COVID test, fears related to possible exposure at the grocery store, and the mental health toll we've observed in our children and aging parents.

Such personal stories could be the key to a transformation in public health communications. As we emerge from this pandemic, we have a unique opportunity to expand meaningful conversations about public health. We can be more approachable and in tune with people's experiences and feelings. We need communication media, like comics, that are highly adaptive, engaging, and accessible. Comics offer explanatory power through the combination of visual and textual elements, and as a storytelling medium, they also encourage connection and empathy.

This is foremost a book for my colleagues in the public health field, who, like me, struggle to engage the public in the work we do. At a time in which misinformation flows freely and even life-saving health information has become politicized, it's more important than ever to find forms of communication that resonate and invite people to connect with issues that profoundly impact their own health and the health of their communities. Public health increasingly focuses on the systems and structures that shape health and addresses the upstream determinants of health. These big-picture views are fundamental to improving health outcomes, but communicating about them to lay audiences so that they become invested in public health efforts is enormously challenging. Storytelling that feels personal and intimate may be more compelling and convincing than our traditional reliance on data charts, brochures, news releases, and fact sheets. Comics, as I will argue, can tell these stories and—as with *No Ordinary Flu*—help people visualize and comprehend how public health concerns are embedded in their own lives.

This book is a comics anthology. It offers examples of how comics can be used as a tool for health communications and also serves as a how-to guide for those interested in making comics for public health or any other public information endeavor. It is by no means a comprehensive volume of graphic public health; there have been many other creative and innovative uses of comics in the field. This collection of comics is limited to the ones that I have worked on as a writer, editor, art director, and/or artist in my professional work for a metropolitan health department or in my private life as an occasional cartoonist. However, this collection doesn't just represent my own individual endeavor. The comics also feature the work of a cadre of talented artists, and I have been fortunate to have them as collaborators.

The first four chapters of this book focus on the use of graphic public health for specific health communication objectives: health literacy, risk communication, health promotion, and advocacy. Each chapter includes a collection of comics followed by my commentary about how comics work for each of these communication functions. I also provide background on the communications strategy used in the development of the comics.

The final chapter is the how-to manual for public health practitioners, communications professionals, and anyone who wants to create comics for public information. It offers details about the logistics of making comics, including developing concepts, establishing the visual style, and working with artists. This chapter considers the unique demands of making comics for public information purposes with explanations of the processes I've used for developing and vetting graphic public health projects. I hope the comics and the resources in this book will encourage others to tell their own graphic public health stories.

1.

Comics for Health Literacy

The Comics

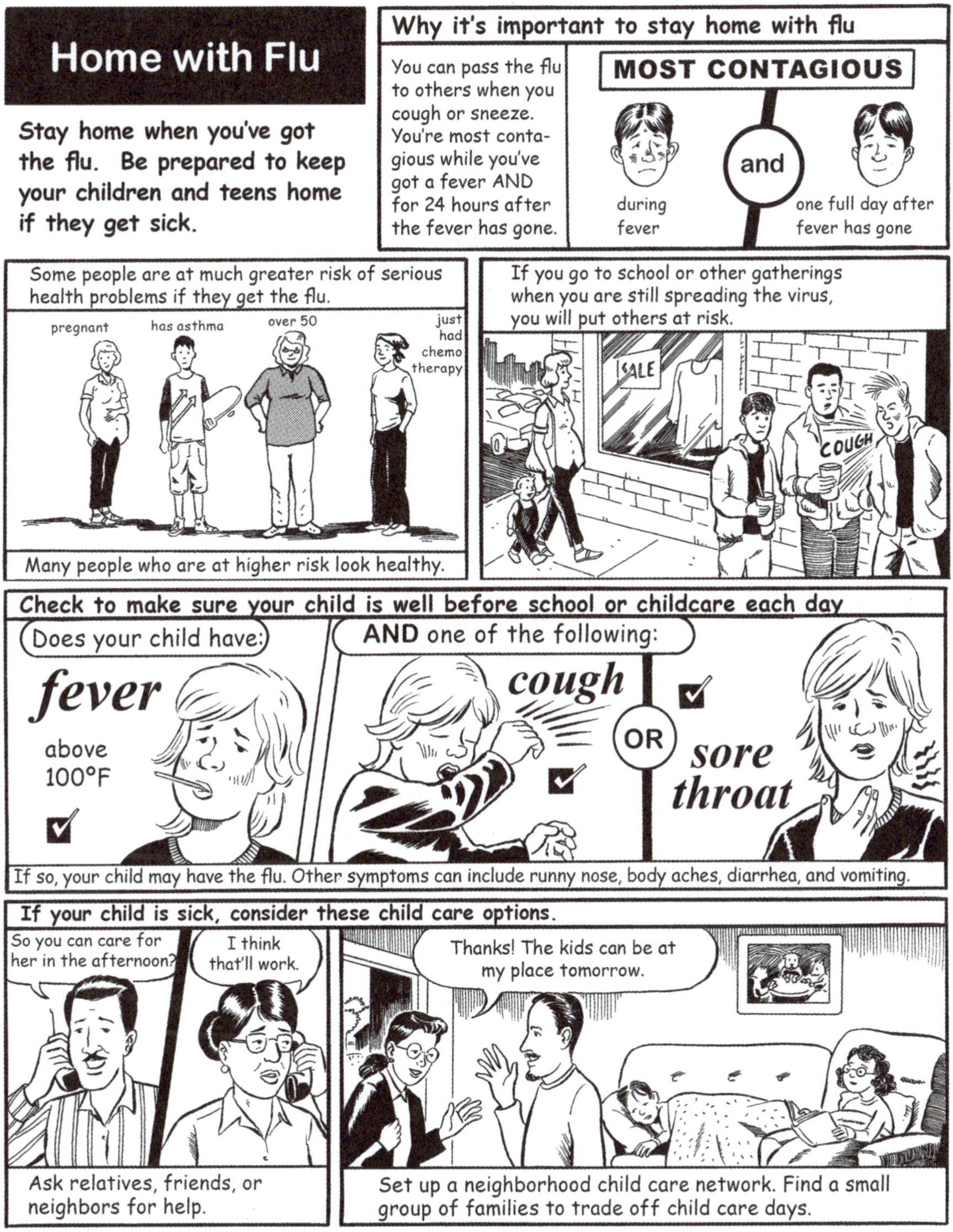
Home with Flu
Stay home when you've got the flu. Be prepared to keep your children and teens home if they get sick.
Why it's important to stay home with flu
You can pass the flu to others when you cough or sneeze. You're most contagious while you've got a fever AND for 24 hours after the fever has gone.
MOST CONTAGIOUS
during fever
and
one full day after fever has gone
Some people are at much greater risk of serious health problems if they get the flu.
pregnant
has asthma
over 50
just had chemo therapy
Many people who are at higher risk look healthy.
If you go to school or other gatherings when you are still spreading the virus, you will put others at risk.
SALE
COUGH
Check to make sure your child is well before school or childcare each day
Does your child have:
fever
above 100°F
AND one of the following:
cough
OR
sore throat
If so, your child may have the flu. Other symptoms can include runny nose, body aches, diarrhea, and vomiting.
If your child is sick, consider these child care options.
So you can care for her in the afternoon?
I think that'll work.
Ask relatives, friends, or neighbors for help.
Thanks! The kids can be at my place tomorrow.
Set up a neighborhood child care network. Find a small group of families to trade off child care days.

APC Advanced Practice Centers

For more information, visit www.kingcounty.gov/health.

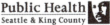

Public Health Seattle & King County

On hot days in King County, many more people have serious health problems.

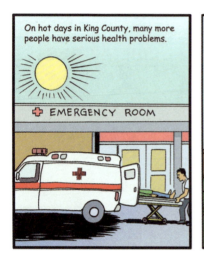

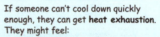

If someone can't cool down quickly enough, they can get **heat exhaustion**. They might feel:
- Muscle cramps
- Dizziness or weakness
- Headache
- Nausea and vomiting

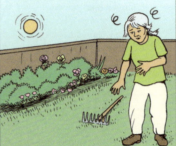

If you have symptoms, move to a cooler place, put your feet up, and drink water.

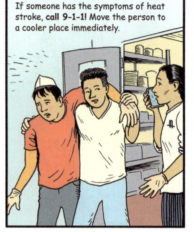

Heat stroke is very serious and can be deadly unless treated immediately. Watch for:
- Extremely high temperature
- Red, hot, and dry skin
- Rapid, strong heartbeat
- Mental confusion and unconsciousness

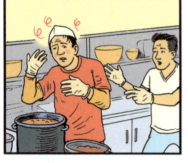

If someone has the symptoms of heat stroke, **call 9-1-1!** Move the person to a cooler place immediately.

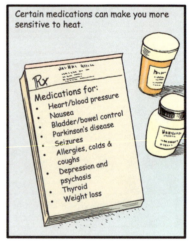

Some people are at greater risk for heart problems, stroke, and kidney failure when it's hot. These are the most common health problems on hot days!

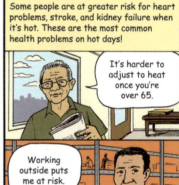

It's harder to adjust to heat once you're over 65.

Working outside puts me at risk.

Some health conditions make it more difficult for your body to cool down.

I have diabetes, so I track my blood sugar levels closely on hot days.

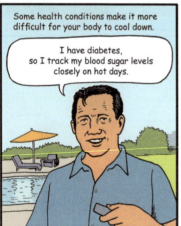

Certain medications can make you more sensitive to heat.

Medications for:
- Heart/blood pressure
- Nausea
- Bladder/bowel control
- Parkinson's disease
- Seizures
- Allergies, colds & coughs
- Depression and psychosis
- Thyroid
- Weight loss

Talk to your doctor or clinician about whether your medications or health conditions put you at greater risk in the heat.

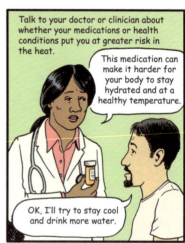

This medication can make it harder for your body to stay hydrated and at a healthy temperature.

OK, I'll try to stay cool and drink more water.

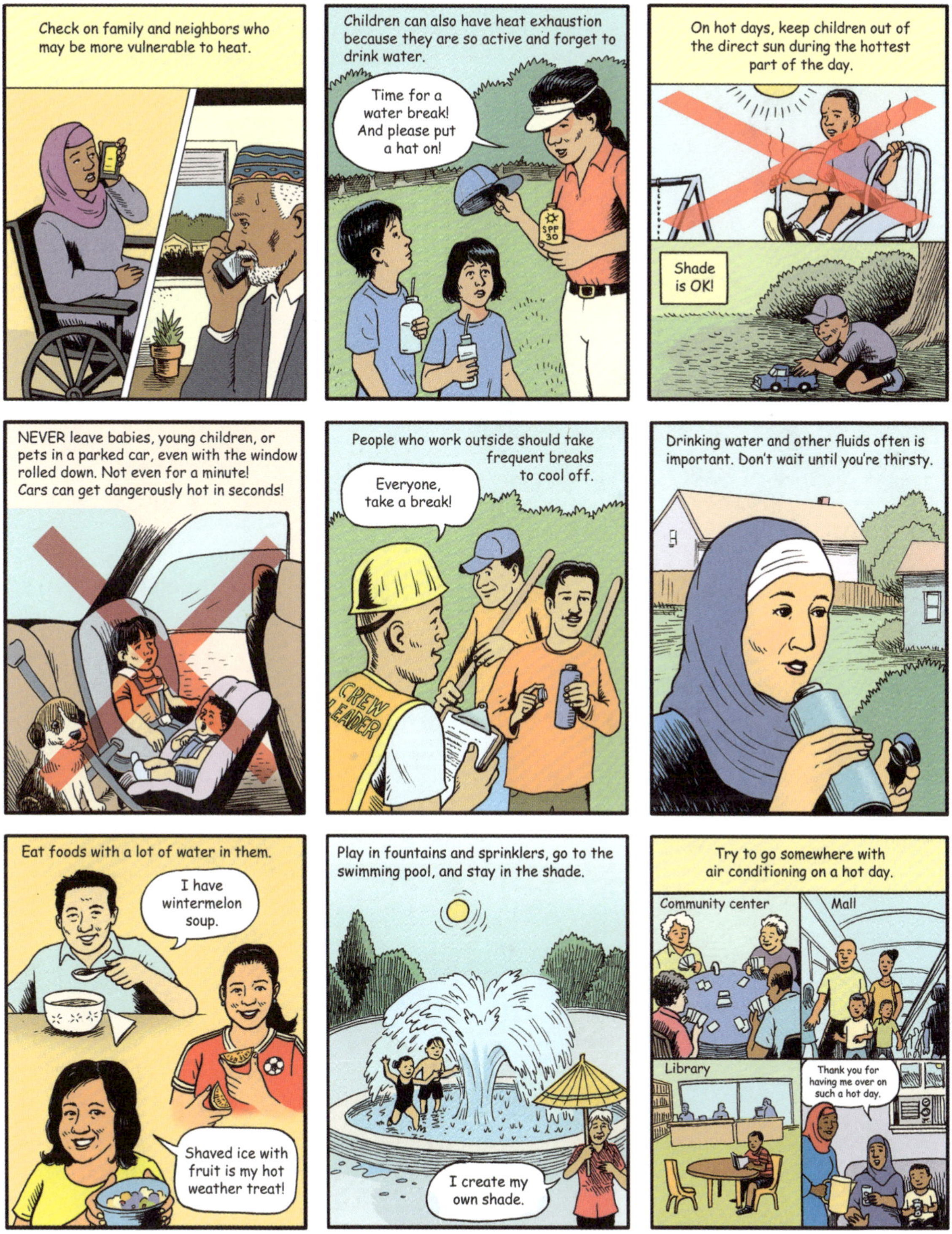

Check on family and neighbors who may be more vulnerable to heat.
Children can also have heat exhaustion because they are so active and forget to drink water.
Time for a water break! And please put a hat on!
SPF 30
On hot days, keep children out of the direct sun during the hottest part of the day.
Shade is OK!
NEVER leave babies, young children, or pets in a parked car, even with the window rolled down. Not even for a minute! Cars can get dangerously hot in seconds!
People who work outside should take frequent breaks to cool off.
Everyone, take a break!
CREW LEADER
Drinking water and other fluids often is important. Don't wait until you're thirsty.
Eat foods with a lot of water in them.
I have wintermelon soup.
Shaved ice with fruit is my hot weather treat!
Play in fountains and sprinklers, go to the swimming pool, and stay in the shade.
I create my own shade.
Try to go somewhere with air conditioning on a hot day.
Community center
Mall
Library
Thank you for having me over on such a hot day.

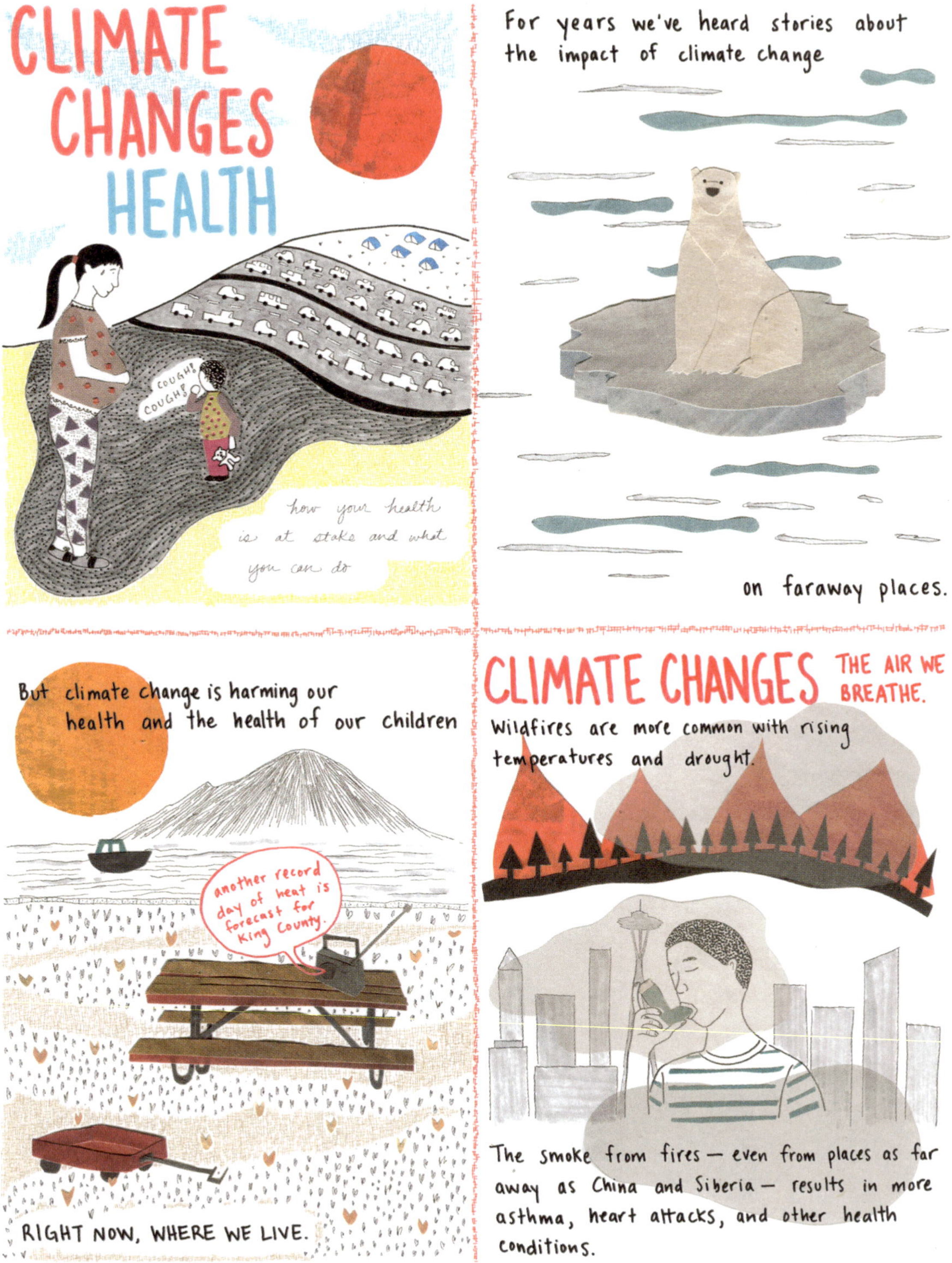
CLIMATE CHANGES HEALTH
COUGH! COUGH!
how your health is at stake and what you can do
For years we've heard stories about the impact of climate change
on faraway places.
But climate change is harming our health and the health of our children
another record day of heat is forecast for King County.
RIGHT NOW, WHERE WE LIVE.
CLIMATE CHANGES THE AIR WE BREATHE.
Wildfires are more common with rising temperatures and drought.
The smoke from fires — even from places as far away as China and Siberia — results in more asthma, heart attacks, and other health conditions.

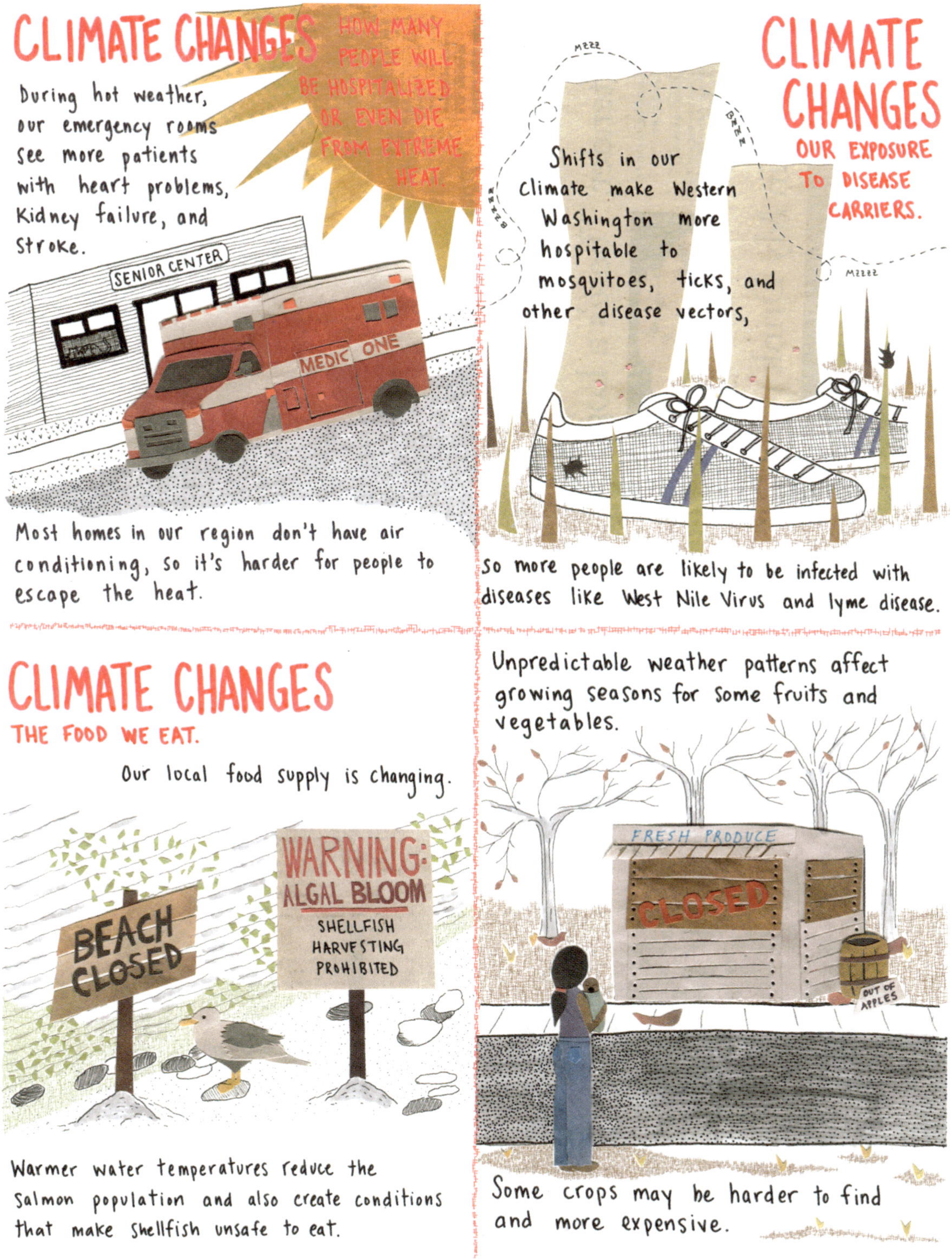
CLIMATE CHANGES
HOW MANY PEOPLE WILL BE HOSPITALIZED OR EVEN DIE FROM EXTREME HEAT.
During hot weather, our emergency rooms see more patients with heart problems, Kidney failure, and stroke.
SENIOR CENTER
MEDIC ONE
Most homes in our region don't have air conditioning, so it's harder for people to escape the heat.
CLIMATE CHANGES
OUR EXPOSURE TO DISEASE CARRIERS.
MZZZ
Shifts in our climate make Western Washington more hospitable to mosquitoes, ticks, and other disease vectors,
MZZZ
so more people are likely to be infected with diseases like West Nile Virus and lyme disease.
CLIMATE CHANGES
THE FOOD WE EAT.
Our local food supply is changing.
BEACH CLOSED
WARNING: ALGAL BLOOM
SHELLFISH HARVESTING PROHIBITED
Warmer water temperatures reduce the salmon population and also create conditions that make shellfish unsafe to eat.
Unpredictable weather patterns affect growing seasons for some fruits and vegetables.
FRESH PRODUCE
CLOSED
OUT OF APPLES
Some crops may be harder to find and more expensive.

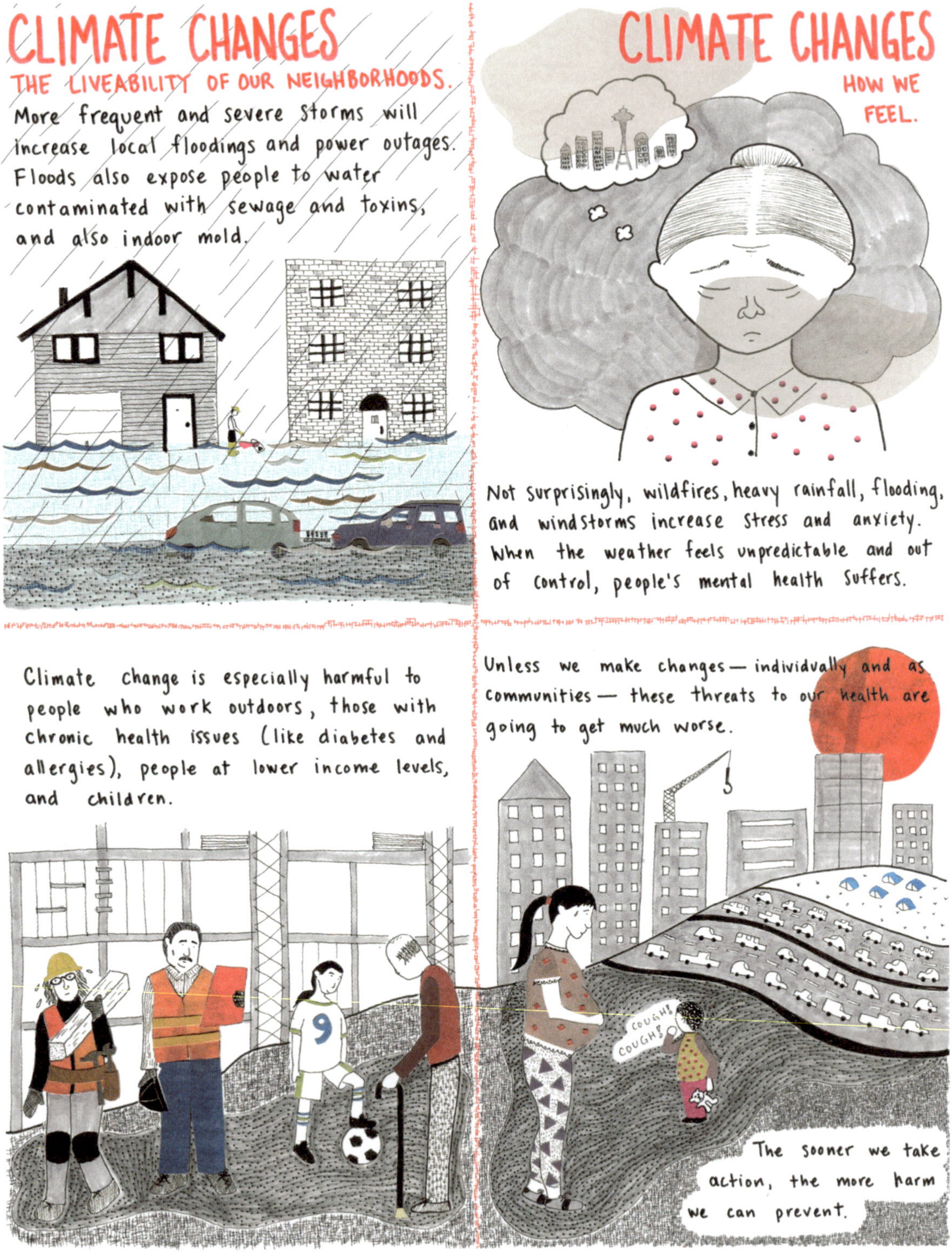
CLIMATE CHANGES
THE LIVEABILITY OF OUR NEIGHBORHOODS.
More frequent and severe storms will increase local floodings and power outages. Floods also expose people to water contaminated with sewage and toxins, and also indoor mold.
CLIMATE CHANGES
HOW WE FEEL.
Not surprisingly, wildfires, heavy rainfall, flooding, and windstorms increase stress and anxiety. When the weather feels unpredictable and out of control, people's mental health suffers.
Climate change is especially harmful to people who work outdoors, those with chronic health issues (like diabetes and allergies), people at lower income levels, and children.
9
Unless we make changes — individually and as communities — these threats to our health are going to get much worse.
COUGH! COUGH!
The sooner we take action, the more harm we can prevent.

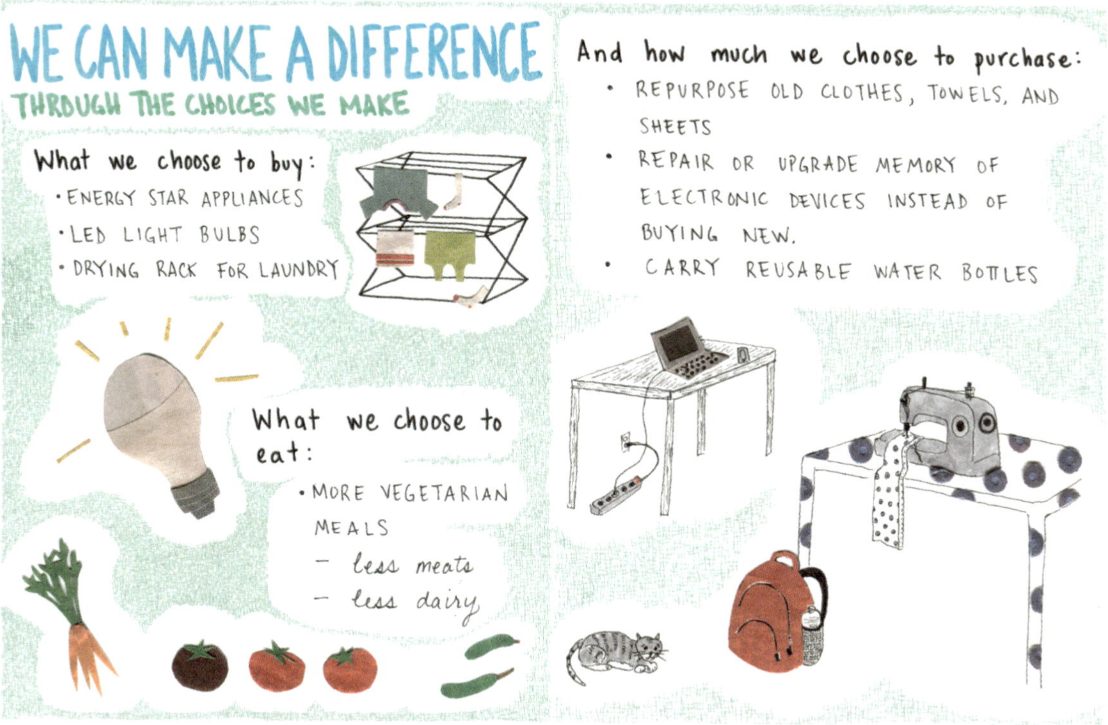
WE CAN MAKE A DIFFERENCE
THROUGH THE CHOICES WE MAKE
What we choose to buy:
• ENERGY STAR APPLIANCES
• LED LIGHT BULBS
• DRYING RACK FOR LAUNDRY
What we choose to eat:
• MORE VEGETARIAN MEALS
– less meats
– less dairy
And how much we choose to purchase:
• REPURPOSE OLD CLOTHES, TOWELS, AND SHEETS
• REPAIR OR UPGRADE MEMORY OF ELECTRONIC DEVICES INSTEAD OF BUYING NEW.
• CARRY REUSABLE WATER BOTTLES

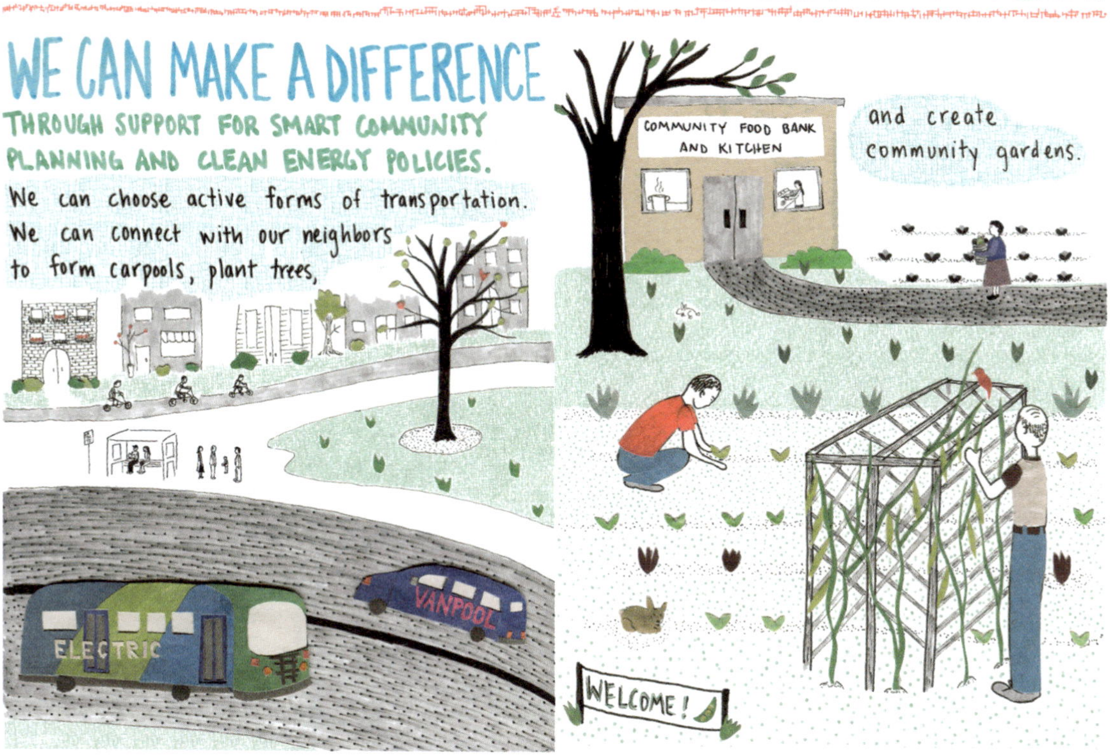
WE CAN MAKE A DIFFERENCE
THROUGH SUPPORT FOR SMART COMMUNITY PLANNING AND CLEAN ENERGY POLICIES.
We can choose active forms of transportation.
We can connect with our neighbors to form carpools, plant trees,
ELECTRIC
VANPOOL
COMMUNITY FOOD BANK AND KITCHEN
and create community gardens.
WELCOME!

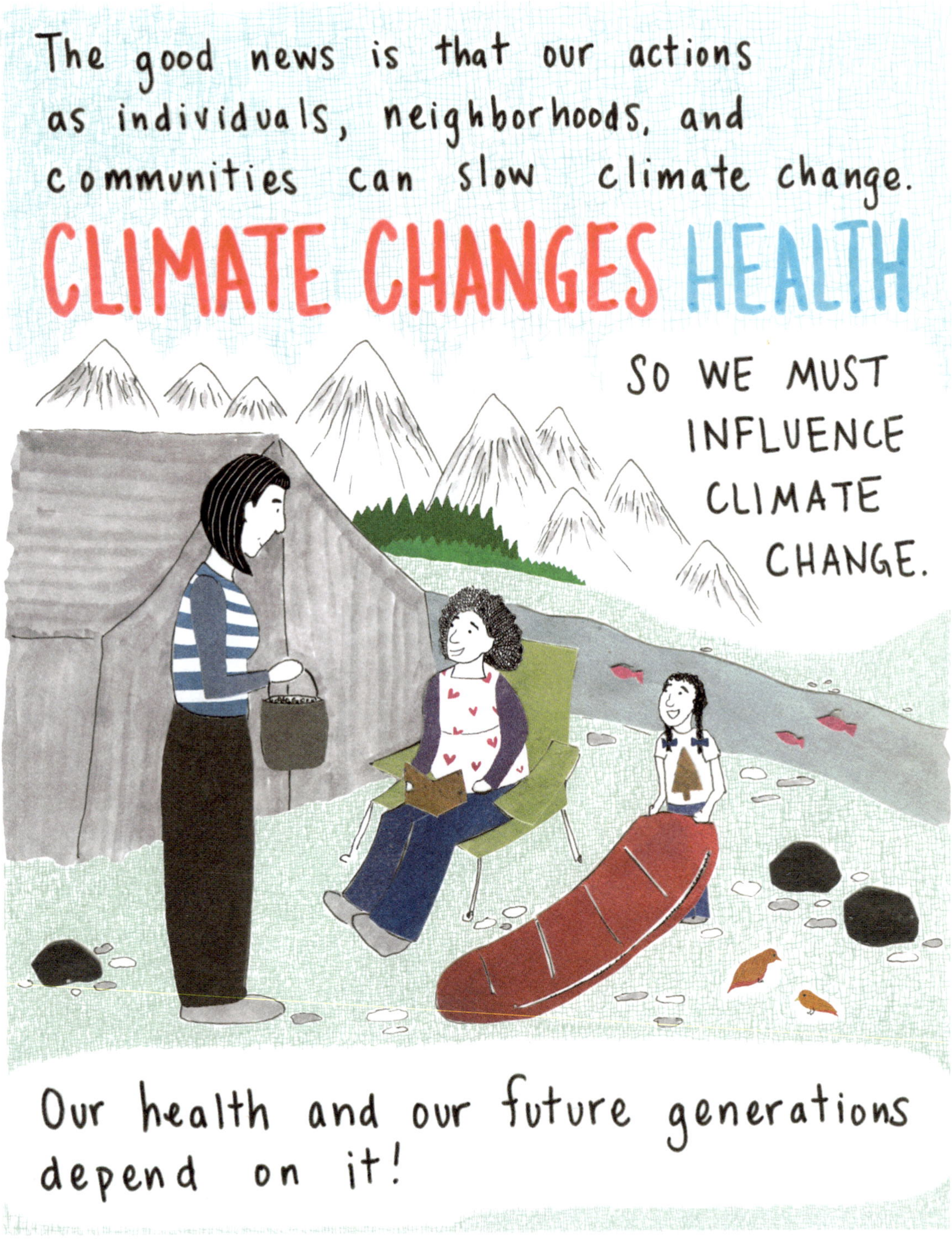
The good news is that our actions as individuals, neighborhoods, and communities can slow climate change.
CLIMATE CHANGES HEALTH
SO WE MUST INFLUENCE CLIMATE CHANGE.
Our health and our future generations depend on it!

Discussion

All of the comics included in this anthology aim to influence how people make decisions that affect their health and the health of the community, whether that's through visually demonstrating health behaviors, or enhancing people's understanding of a complex health issue, or expanding what people consider a public health concern. When comics provoke the reader to contemplate, critically evaluate, or even recognize a public health issue, they work in the service of health literacy.

Advancing health literacy is challenging and complex. Health information is often technical, complicated, and laden with jargon. The impenetrability of some health recommendations can discourage even an avid reader from perusing health education materials, let alone trying to understand them. At the same time, the people we target for health messaging each have their own characteristics and information needs; public health issues may not rank among their main concerns. Health communicators must respond to these factors in their approaches to communication if they want people to access, comprehend, and act upon health messages. They must take into consideration the varying levels of reading ability and numeracy in the general public and the widening gap in science education. They must meet language access needs and ensure relevant communication for diverse audiences, each with distinct health concerns. Communicators must be able to deliver health messages across an ever-growing number of information channels and platforms. Attention spans are shorter in the age of vast digital media, and health messages must compete with expanding sources of misinformation and increasing political rhetoric around public health issues. This complexity calls for new options and approaches.

Comics, I believe, are uniquely well suited to meeting this call. They offer multiple modes for conveying information in a single encounter, and the dynamic visual and textural elements have the potential to garner attention. But the power of comics is more than the explanatory power and attractive visual appeal of illustration and text. Comics offer distinctive possibilities for exploring public health issues through narrative storytelling. They tap into how an issue makes people feel and how it plays out in their realities. Whether or not people engage with public health messages may only minimally be about the clarity of information. They receive a message within the context of their emotional states, their social worlds, and the specifics of their own positionality. Does the message stimulate an emotion? Does it relate to the world as they experience it? The possibilities that comics offer to evoke a response, create connections, and stimulate empathy are the most compelling reasons to use comics for health literacy. By drawing the reader into the social and emotional dynamics of a health message, comics can foster a deeper level of engagement.

Why Comics Work for Health Literacy

The Explanatory Power of Comics

Comics have a unique visual vocabulary that lends itself to conveying specific information and facilitating the construction of meaning, two qualities that make it a powerful medium for promoting health literacy. I became aware of this potential after reading Scott McCloud's groundbreaking work *Understanding Comics*, in which he demonstrates how comics harness multiple elements to communicate, including words, images, flow, moment, and frames. Skillful use of these elements can increase the explanatory power of health information, sharpening its clarity, relaying elements of social context, and amplifying its persuasive quality.

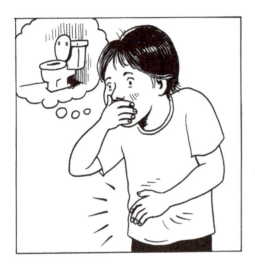

Fig. 1.1. The image alone can powerfully convey the main symptom of norovirus infection. Artwork by David Lasky for "Norovirus Fact Sheet." Courtesy of Public Health—Seattle & King County.

Comics Pack Information Through Pictures

The image is the powerhouse of comics. Even without accompanying text, an image is capable of relaying specific information, such as a demonstration of a desired behavior or an illustration of steps in a process. The density of information packed into a well-planned image can reduce (or in some cases, eliminate) the need for text. For example, without any words, a single panel of a child clutching his stomach and thinking of a toilet can concisely convey the main symptom of norovirus (fig. 1.1).

Comics Add Words for Clarity and Narrative

Images can carry a density of information, but their meanings are still open to interpretation. Images alone do not always result in fidelity of information between sender and receiver, a quality needed when the goal of a piece is to clarify a concept or provide specific instruction. In comics, words can clarify and reinforce the desired meaning as well as expand narrative and expository possibilities.

For example, the images in figure 1.2 convey (without words) that the comic is about illness. By adding just a brief amount of text, the panels in figure 1.3 clearly demonstrate how the flu virus is transmitted.

Writing for comics must be precise and spare to fit into the panel structure. This forced brevity often makes for a better reading experience. Complex sentence structures, passive voice, and wonky jargon frequently obfuscate the key messages in public health writing. When comics are executed well, the image carries much of the meaning,

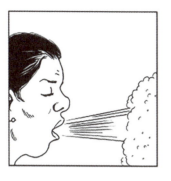
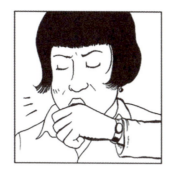
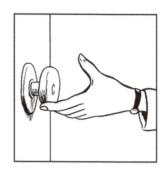

HOW FLU SPREADS

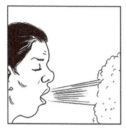
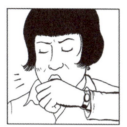
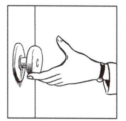

Flu germs spread when people cough, sneeze, or talk.

If flu germs get on hands...

...they can pass the germs to other objects.

Fig. 1.2. Images indicate that this is a message about illness. Artwork by David Lasky for "Flu Fact Sheet." Courtesy of Public Health—Seattle & King County.

Fig. 1.3. Adding text conveys more clearly that this sequence demonstrates how flu spreads. Artwork by David Lasky for "Flu Fact Sheet." Courtesy of Public Health—Seattle & King County.

allowing the text to sparingly fill in information that cannot be derived from images alone. Writing about health within the comics genre challenges the writer to be brief, resulting in lean and focused language that makes information easier to process.

The Sequence in Comics Has Meaning

Unlike other forms of illustration, comics panels can be arranged in sequences that serve an additional informational function. As McCloud notes, panels provide an organization that indicates the passage of time and/or changing of physical space, and they also provide a narrative flow.[1] The comics scholar Hillary Chute has noted that the comics medium's panels and gutters—the spaces between the panels—require the reader to fill in the narrative between the panels to determine how they are connected.[2] The construction of meaning in the gutter can be multidimensional; for instance, reading through a sequence of panels, a reader could interpret the passage of time and also connect what has happened in a concluding panel to be an outcome of what was previously shown.

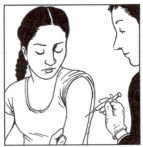
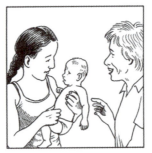

Flu vaccination offers you protection from getting the flu...

...and if you stay well, that protects people who are more vulnerable.

Fig. 1.4. The sequencing of these panels demonstrates how specific behaviors have health outcomes. Artwork by David Lasky for "Flu Fact Sheet." Courtesy of Public Health—Seattle & King County.

For public health purposes, we can use sequence to explain causal relationships, demonstrated in figure 1.3 about the transmission of flu virus. The sequence shows how flu virus transmits indirectly as droplets from coughs and sneezes, and then gets spread from surface contact with objects like doorknobs. To reinforce the importance of the sequence, we used ellipses in the text to propel the reader from panel to panel. By following the flow, the reader can see how easily flu spreads and why hand washing is crucial.

Sequential panels can also be deployed to indicate outcomes of health behaviors. For example, in the first panel in figure 1.4, a patient receives a flu vaccination. In the next panel, because she had the vaccination, the patient can visit an infant and an older adult without risking spreading the flu to her loved ones.

Comics Can Provoke Emotional Responses and Capture Social Contexts

Comics are most successful when the image, words, and sequential elements operate simultaneously to form meaning beyond the literal information presented. Skillful application of these elements can create an emotional response or encourage empathy, and in concert, they have more persuasive power in promoting specific health behaviors.

This is most obvious in a narrative comic with a story line, characters, and dialogue. For example, for *Survivor Tales: Aftershocks*, a comic book for emergency preparedness, we used a real-life story from an American survivor of the Kobe earthquake. The comic book was designed to promote community resilience with the key message that people need to look out for one another during disasters. The protagonist's emotional reactions—as shown through his facial expressions, internal dialogue, and illustrations of the devastation—serve as a model of his concern and care for his neighbors (fig. 1.5).

Comics' various elements can work together for an emotional appeal, even in a nonnarrative, didactic comic about flu prevention. David Lasky and I created a short educational comic that opens this chapter, *Stay Home with Flu*, during the 2009 H1N1 influenza pandemic. At that time, school districts reported that many sick children were coming to school despite public health messaging that urged caregivers to keep

We were lucky. We lived on a part of an island where there wasn't a lot of damage. But we could see that it was much worse elsewhere in Kobe.
In some places, it looked like a giant had ripped up the ground.
Are you OK, Mrs. Hayashi?
Well, a falling book smashed my glasses, and stuff fell every-where. But I'm OK.
Everyone pitched in to help each other.

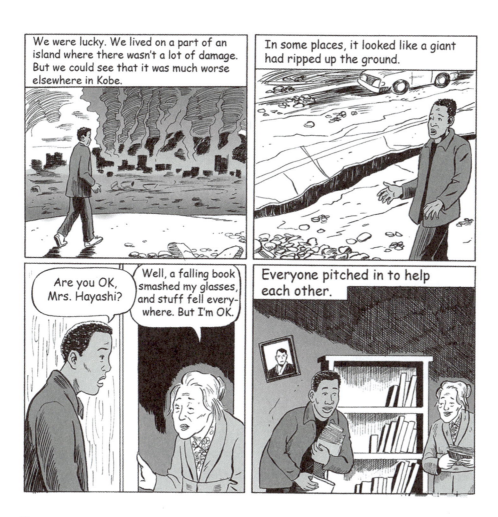

Fig. 1.5. A comic about the aftermath of the Kobe earthquake drew upon the character's emotional reactions to reinforce the need for neighbors to help one another—a key factor in community resilience. Artwork by David Lasky for *Survivor Tales: Aftershocks*. Courtesy of Public Health—Seattle & King County.

kids home to help them recover. We decided to try a different angle, emphasizing staying home to prevent spreading flu to those most vulnerable to hospitalization.

Stay Home with Flu shows the kinds of people who are most vulnerable to the most serious illness from flu. The words clarify why they are more vulnerable, and through a combination of words and images, the comic explains that they might not look more susceptible. The drawings of these high-risk people, with their outward gaze and friendly demeanor, help make an empathetic connection with the reader.

Sequence is at play in a variety of ways. In the first panel, we meet the pregnant woman as someone more vulnerable to flu. In the second panel, she enters the space occupied by someone sick with flu, and we can anticipate her exposure as we mentally

follow the logical flow of her moving through the space in the panel. Because we have already met her and know her vulnerability, we may feel a stronger emotional pull as she is put at risk by ill people.

The examples from *Stay Home with Flu* and *Survivor Tales: Aftershocks* show how the comics genre can also incorporate social dynamics, adding dimension to health communication. Social dynamics can include how characters react to situations or one another, with consideration of facial expressions and gestures that serve the desired message and tap into an appropriate emotion. For example, in comics that include advice to get vaccinated, we were intentional in depicting calm expressions on the patients and reassuring ones on the clinicians (fig. 1.6).

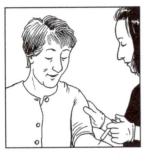

The best way to prevent the flu is to get a flu vaccine every year.

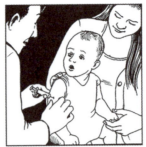

Health experts recommend the vaccine for all people 6 months and older.

Fig. 1.6. The calm, positive facial expressions shown on both the vaccinators and the patients were designed to promote confidence in vaccination and reduce anxiety. Artwork by David Lasky for "Flu Fact Sheet." Courtesy of Public Health—Seattle & King County.

Comics Can Reflect Lived Experience

Comics' ability to convey social contexts and interactions are particularly useful in health literacy efforts targeted at specific audiences. In the health department in King County, Washington, we have been using comics in response to input from advocates and partners in immigrant and refugee groups who call for health communications with less text, more pictorial content, and more reflection of their communities. Comics can literally reflect the target audiences by including aspects of specific communities visually. This is not just a demonstration of respect or a mechanism to attract the communities' attention through representation (though that is part of the intention). Health information is more relevant when the reader sees people, places, and cultural practices that are familiar.

Stay Safe in the Heat, one of the comics at the opening of this chapter, was designed as a mini-comic for specific communities of color living in south King County, Washington. Research by the University of Washington's Occupational and Environmental Health program indicated that proportionally, on hot days, more people from these largely immigrant communities came into emergency rooms suffering from cardiac arrest, kidney failure, and stroke. We worked with this UW program to develop a comic to create more awareness of these health impacts from heat, specific risk factors, and what people can do to prevent heat illness. Focus groups in the affected demographics helped us understand perceptions about health risks from hot weather and what practices

ĐẢM BẢO AN TOÀN KHI TRỜI NÓNG
Một số người có nguy cơ mắc các bệnh về tim, đột quỵ và suy thận cao hơn khi trời nóng. Đây là các bệnh phổ biến nhất vào những ngày nóng bức!
Việc quen khí hậu nóng sẽ khó khăn hơn khi bạn 65 tuổi trở lên.
Làm việc ở ngoài trời cũng khiến cho tôi gặp nguy cơ bị cảm nhiệt.
Một vài tình trạng sức khỏe khiến cơ thể của bạn khó giảm nhiệt độ hơn.
Người đàn ông tuổi trung niên một Đảo của Thái Bình Dương nói: "Tôi bị bệnh tiểu đường, vì vậy tôi phải theo dõi mức đường huyết của mình vào những ngày thời tiết nóng.
Hãy hỏi bác sĩ hoặc nhà cung cấp dịch vụ chăm sóc sức khỏe xem các loại thuốc của bạn hoặc tình trạng sức khỏe có khiến bạn dễ mắc bệnh hơn khi trời nóng hay không.
Thuốc này có thể làm cho cơ thể của bạn khó tích nước và duy trì nhiệt độ tốt cho sức khỏe hơn.
Vậy thì tôi sẽ cố gắng giữ cơ thể mát mẻ và uống nhiều nước hơn.
Những người làm việc ngoài trời nên thường xuyên nghỉ ngơi để làm mát cơ thể.
Mọi người, hãy nghỉ giải lao!
CREW LEADER
Hãy ăn các thực phẩm chứa nhiều nước.
Tôi ăn canh bí đao.
Ăn hoa quả kèm đá bào là giải pháp của tôi khi thời tiết nóng bức!
Hãy đảm bảo an toàn cho gia đình và những người xung quanh bạn -- những người dễ nhạy cảm với nhiệt hơn.
KHÔNG BAO GIỜ để trẻ sơ sinh, trẻ nhỏ, hoặc thú nuôi trong một chiếc xe đang đậu, ngay cả với các cửa sổ đã được quay xuống. Không làm như vậy dù chỉ trong một phút! Xe hơi có thể nóng rất nhanh chỉ trong vài giây!
Để biết thêm thông tin:
www.kingcounty.gov/beattheheat
Made possible with funding by the Centers for Disease Control & Prevention, Office of Public Health Preparedness and Response, and University of Washington Department of Environmental and Occupational Health Sciences
DEPARTMENT OF ENVIRONMENTAL & OCCUPATIONAL HEALTH SCIENCES
UNIVERSITY of WASHINGTON
School of Public Health
Public Health
Seattle & King County

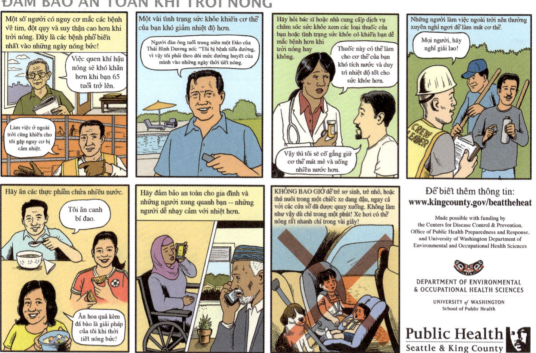

Fig. 1.7. Comics are well suited for publication in community and multilingual newspapers, such as this version of *Stay Safe in the Heat* printed in a Vietnamese newspaper. Artwork by David Lasky. Courtesy of Public Health—Seattle & King County.

specific communities use to keep cool. Community input and reference photos of people in the target communities also informed the development of the comic. The protective behaviors shown—such as drinking winter melon soup or carrying an umbrella for shade—came from community interviews. Community members also reviewed early drafts to make sure that the comic was appealing and contained clear key messages, accurate depictions, actionable tips, and quality translations.

Comics help circumvent barriers to health information that members of non-English language communities frequently encounter. When images carry much of the meaning, health information requires fewer words and allows for simpler syntax. The simpler text in English makes comics easier to read and also results in less expensive and higher-quality translation into other languages. We could afford to translate *Stay Safe in the Heat*, for example, into the ten languages of target communities because the word count was relatively low. Much like traditional comic strips, the comics also adapted well to print media that are widely read within many language communities, such as the Vietnamese-language newspapers that circulate in the Seattle region (fig. 1.7).

Compared to pictograms and icons—other visuals frequently used in health outreach materials—comics provide more context that facilitates understanding. Health information in comics can be drawn more precisely, in a more lifelike manner, making the meaning less ambiguous. In contrast, icons and pictograms are not truly universal; people of different backgrounds interpret them in different ways. Comics are also open to interpretation, but they can more accurately and minutely depict the desired health behavior. And when people see images in comics that reflect their reality, they may find it easier to visualize themselves doing the illustrated health behaviors.

Comics for Public Health Literacy

The use of comics for health literacy discussed so far relates to individual health decisions and behaviors. Within the public health discipline, we are increasingly looking beyond the role of the individual to focus attention on the populations, systems, and institutions that create the conditions for health. "Public health literacy" takes the notion of health literacy further to address the degree to which people comprehend and appreciate how health issues affect them, their communities, and society as a whole.[3] Public health literacy efforts aim to engage more stakeholders in the mission of public health and address the social and environmental determinants of health.[4]

However, it's not easy to make complex discussions about the upstream, structural factors in public health inviting and accessible. Public health conversations about systems change and the social determinants of health can feel academic and removed from the very people at the heart of the issues. As a communication tool, comics can help personalize policy issues, center the community in the discussion, and provide a storytelling thread to help readers piece the complexity together (see more discussion in chapter 4, "Comics for Advocacy and Activism").

Comics can also frame issues as public health concerns. For example, climate change is a pressing public health issue, regarded by many in the field as one of the highest priorities. But members of the general public—and even some of the public health workforce—often don't view it as a health issue. In the Puget Sound region, where I live, climate change is a top policy issue, but dialogue tends to focus on greenhouse gas emissions, carbon footprints, and energy goals. To center the impact of climate change on *people* and provide incentives to slow climate change, I collaborated with colleagues working at the intersection of climate change and health to make a mini-comic.

This group wanted to reach segments of the public who would have the greatest ability to make personal changes to slow the rate of climate change. The mini-comic, *Climate Changes Health*, targeted parents in higher-income demographic groups who tend to have the largest carbon footprint, in terms of their energy use and consumption patterns, and also have the means to prevent further harm to the environment. In this respect, the comic aimed to promote consumption choices that minimize impact on the environment and to increase support for clean-energy policies. The comic also defines climate change as an urgent public health issue and makes concrete the impact of climate change on communicable disease transmission, chronic health conditions, environmental health, and mental health.

Artist Mita Mahato, known for her beautiful cut-paper comics on environmental topics, created the visual style that reinforced the health messages in *Climate Changes Health*. The layered textures of inking and semi-translucent paper evoke the scratchiness of dry grass and the oppressiveness of wildfire smoke. The hand-lettering makes the mini-comic feel personal, like thoughts jotted down by a friend. In the final panels, where the comic shows that people can choose to consume less and reuse and repair what they have, her cut-paper and hand-inking reflect the DIY nature of the recommendations. Mahato's illustrations were instrumental to our strategy; knowing that some people in the target demographic have lost interest in climate change, we aimed to draw them in with visuals too lovely to ignore.

A Role for Comics to Advance the Public Health Mission

Comics for public health literacy is one of the most exciting applications of graphic public health. Public health literacy aims to shift public understanding of health issues to consider how social, political, and environmental pressures reverberate in the health of our communities. If we are to succeed in making this shift and engaging people broadly as stakeholders in public health efforts, we need powerful communication tools, ones that can pull people in with strong storytelling, emotional impact, and striking visuals. Comics can be a valuable part of the public health literacy arsenal, as I discuss in greater depth in chapter 5, "Making Comics for Public Health and Public Information." Already there have been great comics that advance public health literacy by cartoonists such as Whit Taylor, Josh Neufeld, and Malaka Gharib, as well as my collaborators in this volume.[5] I'm looking forward to seeing this use of comics grow.

Comics to Advance Multiple Levels of Health Literacy

At the most basic, functional level of health literacy, comics can convey health information and have been shown to make complex information more understandable, increase knowledge of health risks, and influence healthy choices.[6] For example, when David Lasky and I created educational comics presenting information about norovirus, tuberculosis, and other communicable diseases, we conducted formative testing with target audiences of Asian, Latinx, and East African immigrants. Most respondents reported that the comics made the information easier to understand, and they could explain the protective actions described in the comics.

Improving access to health information is an important and practical use of comics. The explanatory power and visual appeal of comics can help meet calls for the public health field to ensure that health information is accessible and comprehensible to people with diverse informational needs. In addition to the comics shown in this chapter, chapter 2, "Comics for Risk Communication," includes examples of comics designed to convey critical health messages for functional health literacy purposes.

But health literacy involves more than just providing information, and the strength of comics for public health extends well beyond an informative function. More interactive levels of health literacy are possible when there is a dynamic interaction with readers as they actively interpret the communication and apply health messages according to their own unique understandings and circumstances. In a special issue of the journal *Critical Inquiry* devoted to comics and media, Hillary Chute and Patrick Jagoda argue that the interplay between comics and the reader generates robust reader involvement.[7] The specific visual vocabulary of comics—with its panels, gutters, and text bubbles, its juxtapositions of text and images, and its jumps in time and sequence—requires effort on the reader's part to make sense of what happens from panel to panel. While comics can make aspects of information salient and accessible, as Chute notes, piecing together the meaning from the dynamic elements requires a high degree of engagement.[8] As Scott McCloud puts it, the secret language of comics is economical and dense at the same time.[9]

Comics may support interactive health literacy when they facilitate people's ability to act on what they know about health, such as increasing motivation or feelings of self-confidence in performing healthy behaviors or making health decisions.[10] Chapter 3, "Comics for Health Promotion," offers examples of graphic public health used in campaigns that bridge functional health literacy with elements of interactive health literacy.

At a higher level, the activity required by the reader in interpreting comics, particularly narrative comics, may have the potential to activate what Don Nutbeam and Susie Sykes et al. refer to as critical health literacy, in which people become more aware and involved in health issues, participating in critical dialogue and decision making about their personal and community health.[11] For example, Sarah McNicol conducted in-depth interviews with people after they had read educational comics that related to health conditions they or their loved ones were experiencing. They reported that the comics evoked empathy and, on occasion, strong emotional responses of concern and even distress. The situations shown resonated with their own experiences, and some interviewees felt that the comics helped them relate to, respond to, and remember the information better than if it had been offered in a more abstract way. Significantly, the interviewees in McNicol's study also described how the visual metaphors used in the comics provided avenues for them to understand their own health conditions from other perspectives, prompting them to reflect on and reexamine their own understandings.[12]

Readers' greater involvement in interpreting the narrative forms of comics suggests that storytelling or journalism using comics, in concert with the emotional pull of the medium, could promote critical health literacy by encouraging reflection and critical perspectives on complex public health issues. Digesting information through narrative comics may stimulate greater insight into health issues than less personal health recommendations or "neutral" health information. Chapter 2 and chapter 4 offer story-driven comics and comics journalism about public health disasters, health care access, and other public issues as examples of how narrative comics can be used to promote critical health literacy.

2.

Comics for Risk Communication

The Comics

Pandemic Comics

Emergency Preparedness Comics

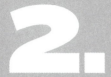

IN 1918, A TERRIBLE DISEASE RANSACKED THE GLOBE,
THE MOST DEADLY DISEASE OUTBREAK IN MODERN HISTORY.
THE DISEASE WAS INFLUENZA, BUT IT WAS...

NO
ORDINARY
FLU

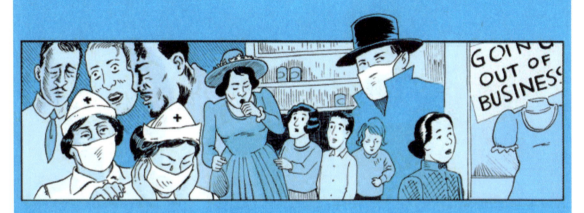

ALSO IN THIS ISSUE:
HOW YOU CAN PREPARE
FOR THE CURRENT
PANDEMIC THREAT

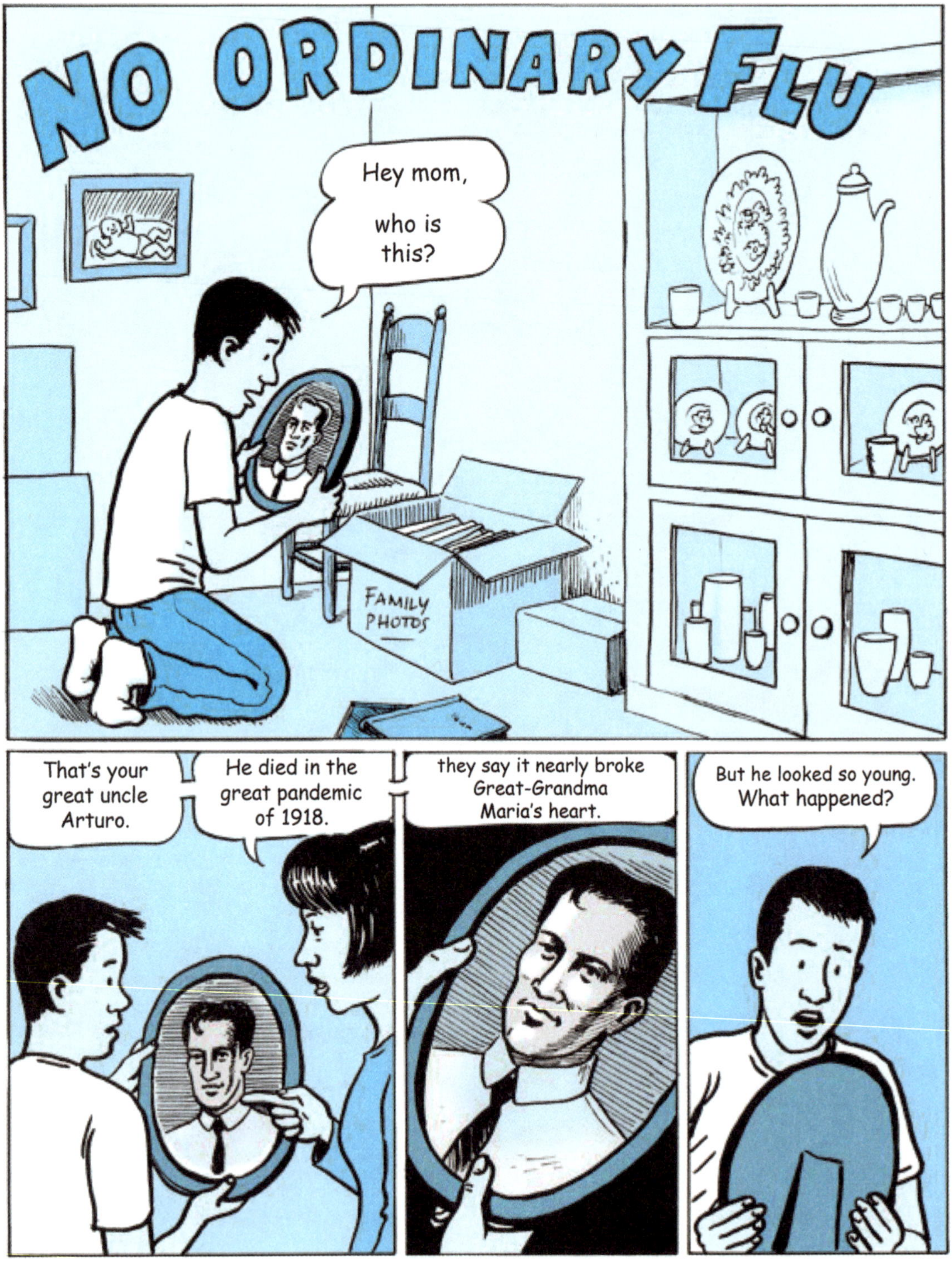
NO ORDINARY FLU
Hey mom,
who is this?
FAMILY PHOTOS
That's your great uncle Arturo.
He died in the great pandemic of 1918.
they say it nearly broke Great-Grandma Maria's heart.
But he looked so young. What happened?

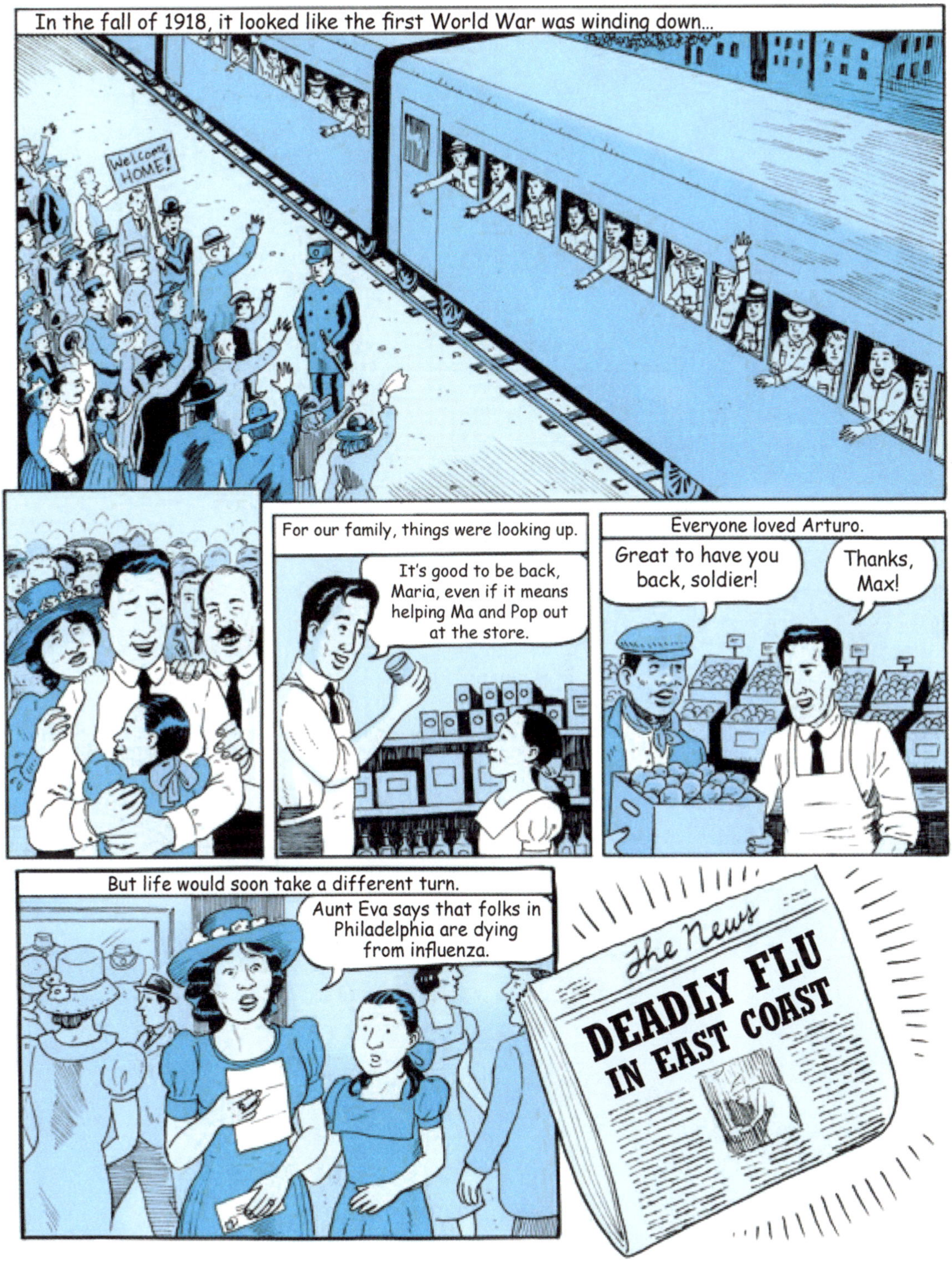
In the fall of 1918, it looked like the first World War was winding down...
Welcome HOME!
For our family, things were looking up.
It's good to be back, Maria, even if it means helping Ma and Pop out at the store.
Everyone loved Arturo.
Great to have you back, soldier!
Thanks, Max!
But life would soon take a different turn.
Aunt Eva says that folks in Philadelphia are dying from influenza.
The News
DEADLY FLU IN EAST COAST

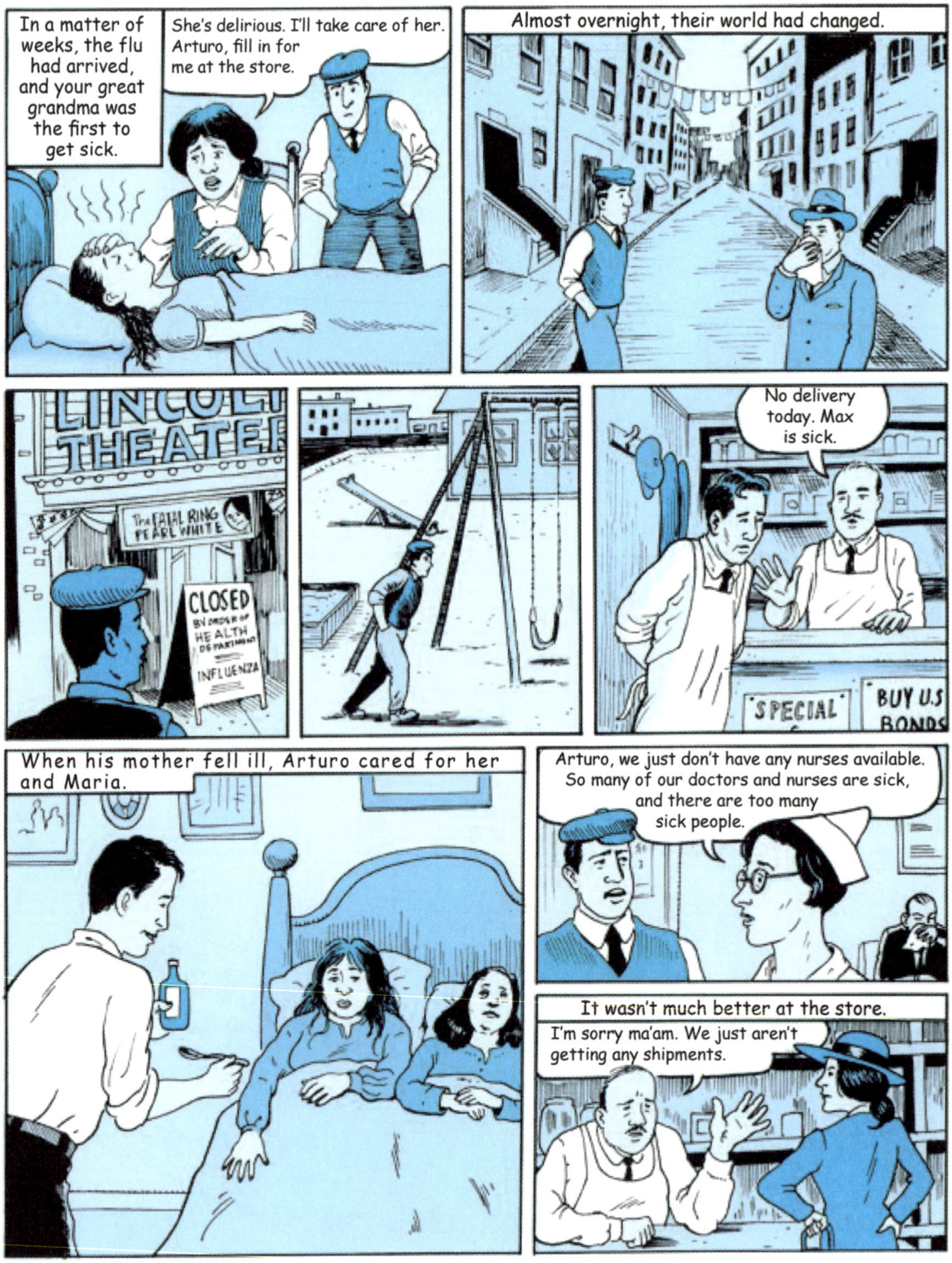
In a matter of weeks, the flu had arrived, and your great grandma was the first to get sick.
She's delirious. I'll take care of her. Arturo, fill in for me at the store.
Almost overnight, their world had changed.
LINCOL
THEATE
The FATAL RING
PEARL WHITE
CLOSED
BY ORDER OF
HEALTH
DEPARTMENT
INFLUENZA
No delivery today. Max is sick.
SPECIAL
BUY U.S
BONDS
When his mother fell ill, Arturo cared for her and Maria.
Arturo, we just don't have any nurses available. So many of our doctors and nurses are sick, and there are too many sick people.
It wasn't much better at the store.
I'm sorry ma'am. We just aren't getting any shipments.

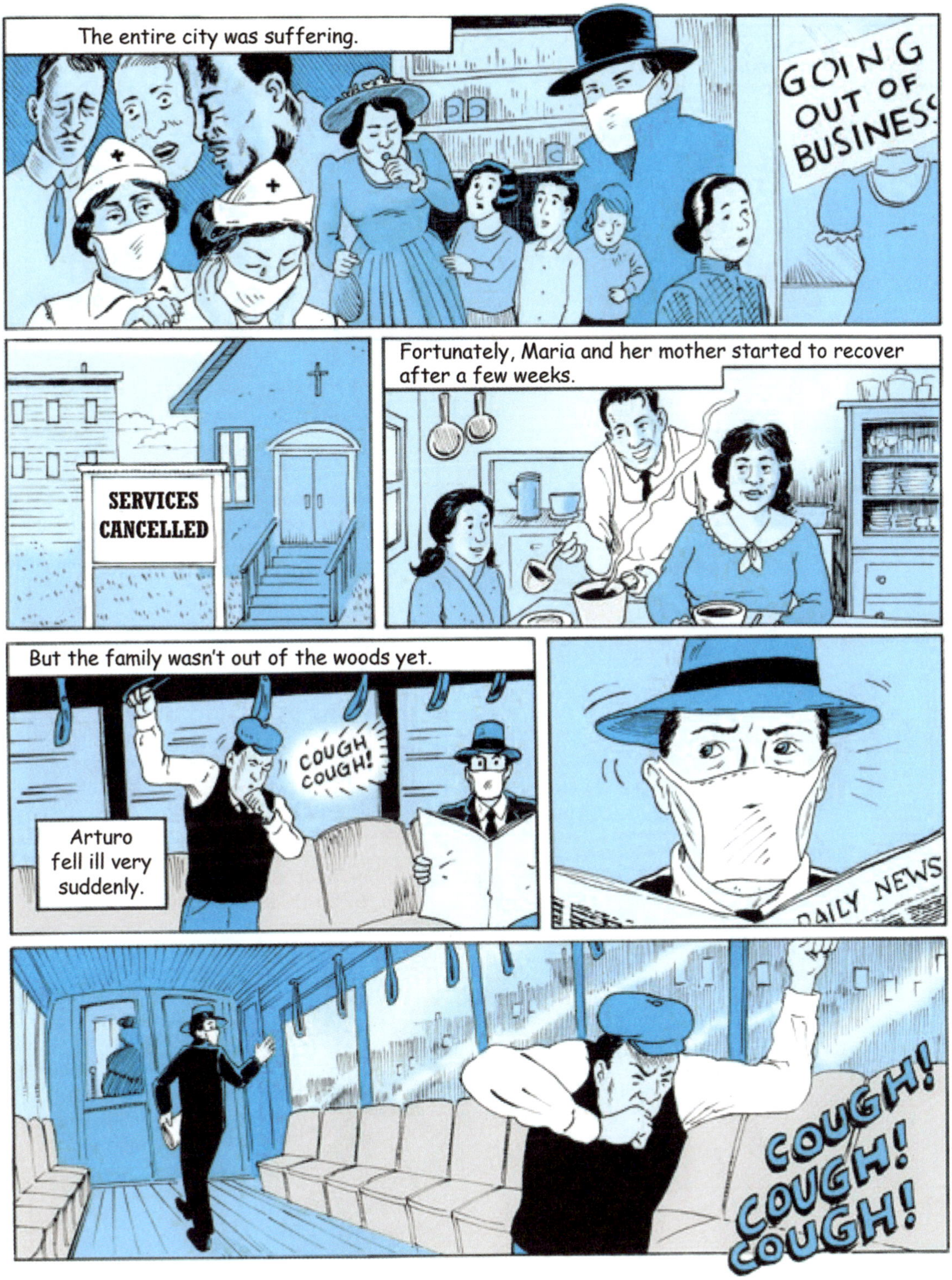

The entire city was suffering.
GOING OUT OF BUSINESS
SERVICES CANCELLED
Fortunately, Maria and her mother started to recover after a few weeks.
But the family wasn't out of the woods yet.
Arturo fell ill very suddenly.
COUGH COUGH!
DAILY NEWS
COUGH! COUGH! COUGH!

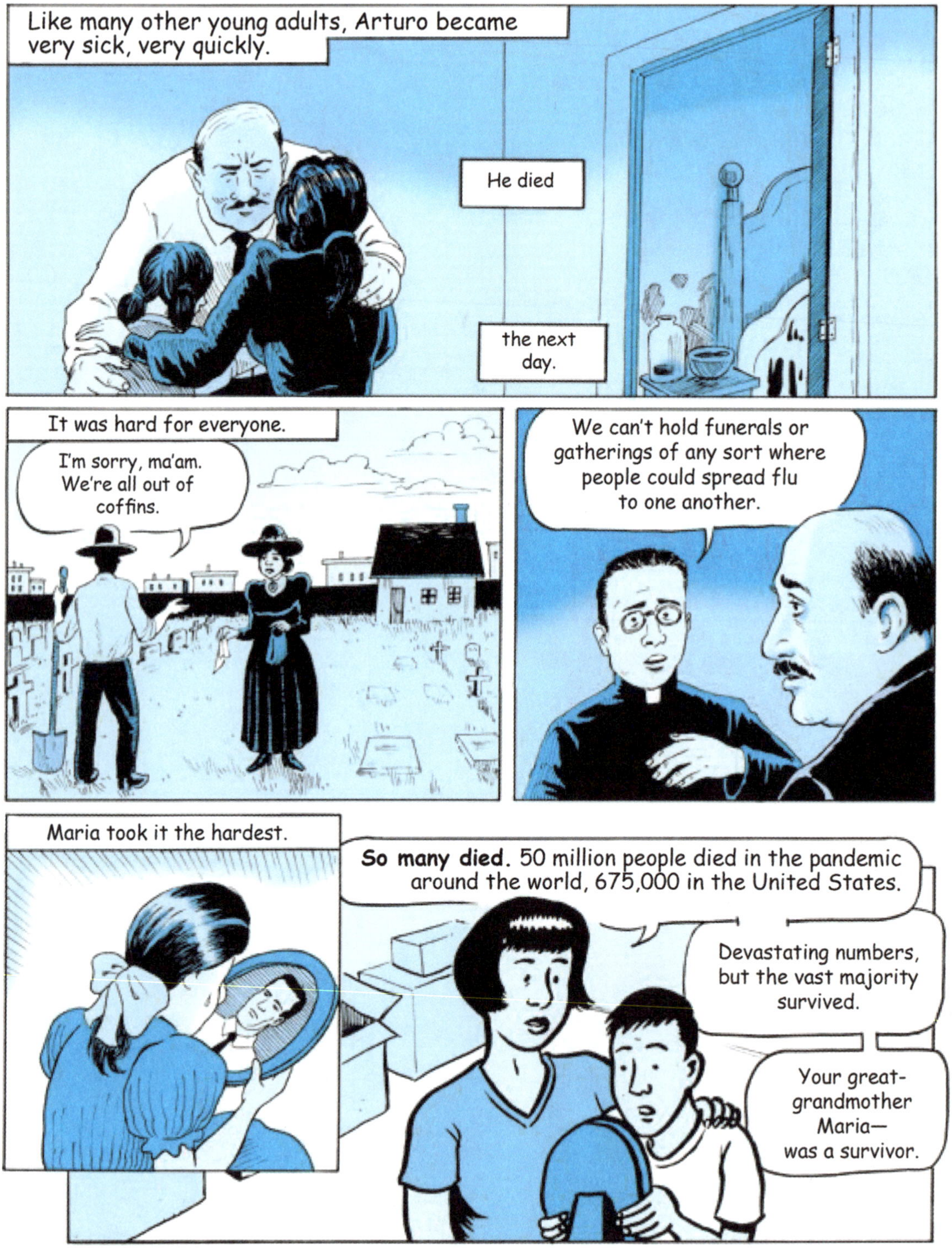
Like many other young adults, Arturo became very sick, very quickly.
He died
the next day.
It was hard for everyone.
I'm sorry, ma'am. We're all out of coffins.
We can't hold funerals or gatherings of any sort where people could spread flu to one another.
Maria took it the hardest.
So many died. 50 million people died in the pandemic around the world, 675,000 in the United States.
Devastating numbers, but the vast majority survived.
Your great-grandmother Maria—was a survivor.

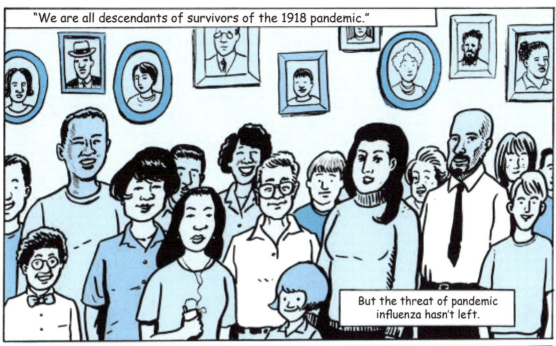

"We are all descendants of survivors of the 1918 pandemic."

But the threat of pandemic influenza hasn't left.

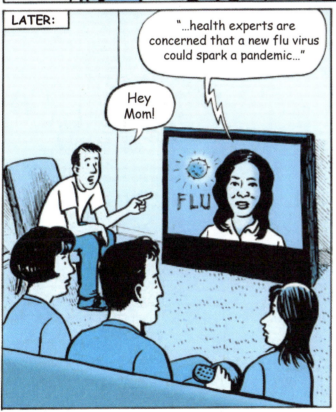

LATER:

"...health experts are concerned that a new flu virus could spark a pandemic..."

Hey Mom!

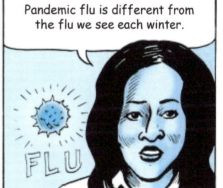

Pandemic flu is different from the flu we see each winter.

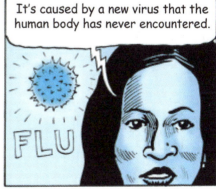

It's caused by a new virus that the human body has never encountered.

Our bodies will have trouble fighting a new flu virus.

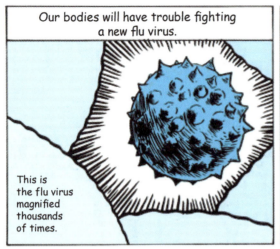

This is the flu virus magnified thousands of times.

Unlike the flu we see each winter, there is no pandemic flu vaccine at this time.

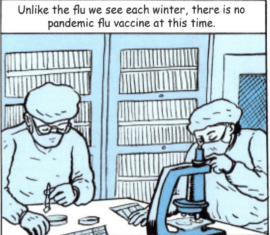

A pandemic virus would spread quickly through contact between people.

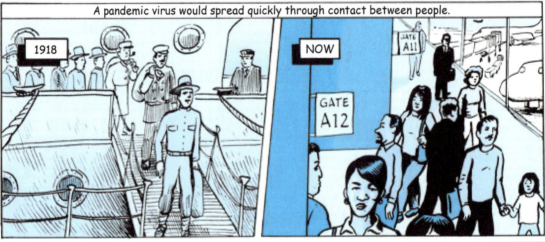

1918

NOW

GATE A11

GATE A12

Pandemic flu will spread to every corner of the world. Everywhere, everyday life will change.

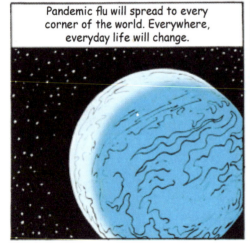

To slow the spread disease, schools and daycares may close.

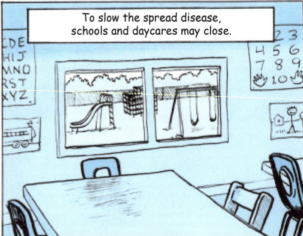

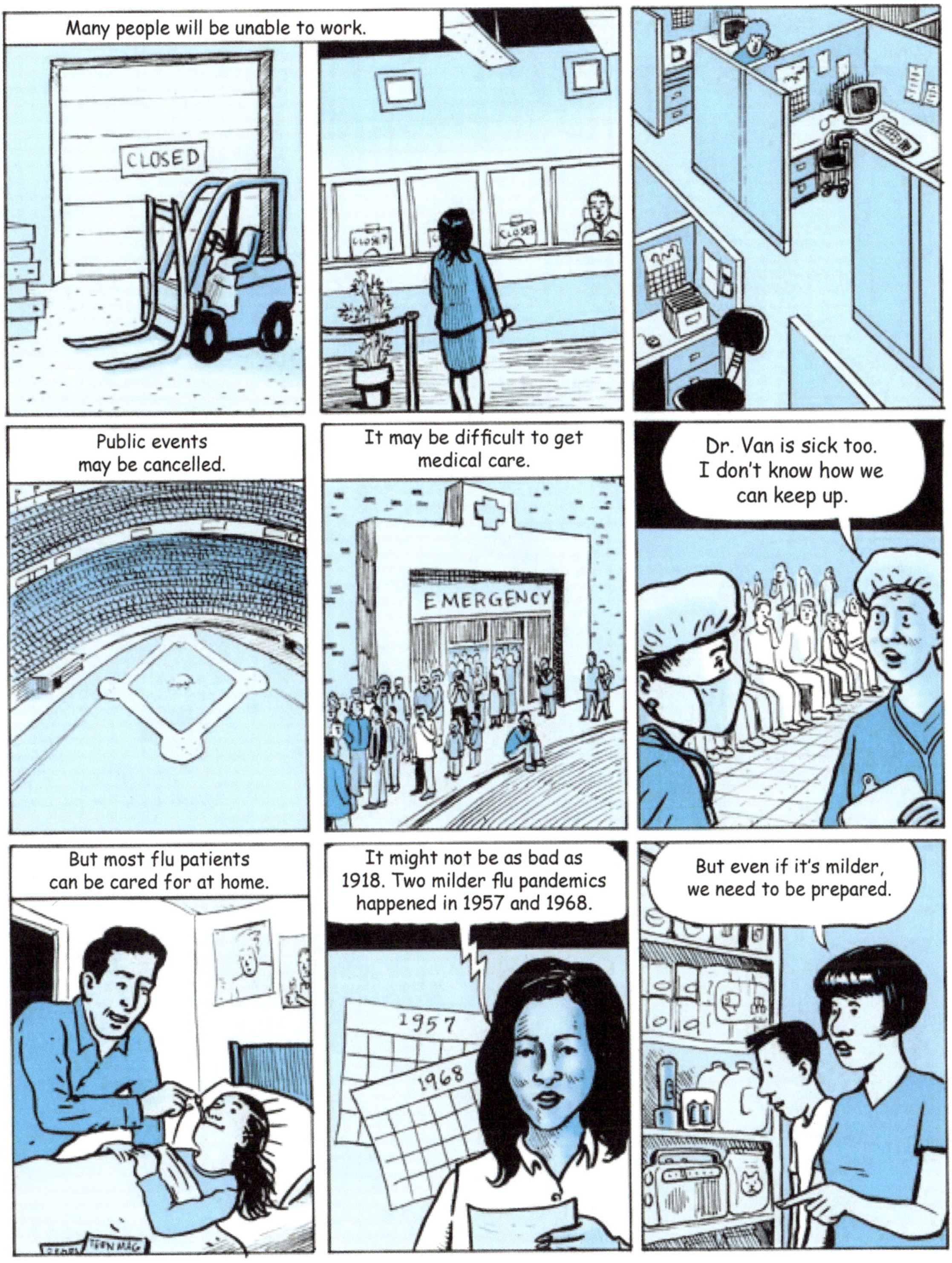
Many people will be unable to work.
CLOSED
CLOSED
CLOSED
Public events may be cancelled.
It may be difficult to get medical care.
EMERGENCY
Dr. Van is sick too. I don't know how we can keep up.
But most flu patients can be cared for at home.
TEEN MAG
It might not be as bad as 1918. Two milder flu pandemics happened in 1957 and 1968.
1957
1968
But even if it's milder, we need to be prepared.

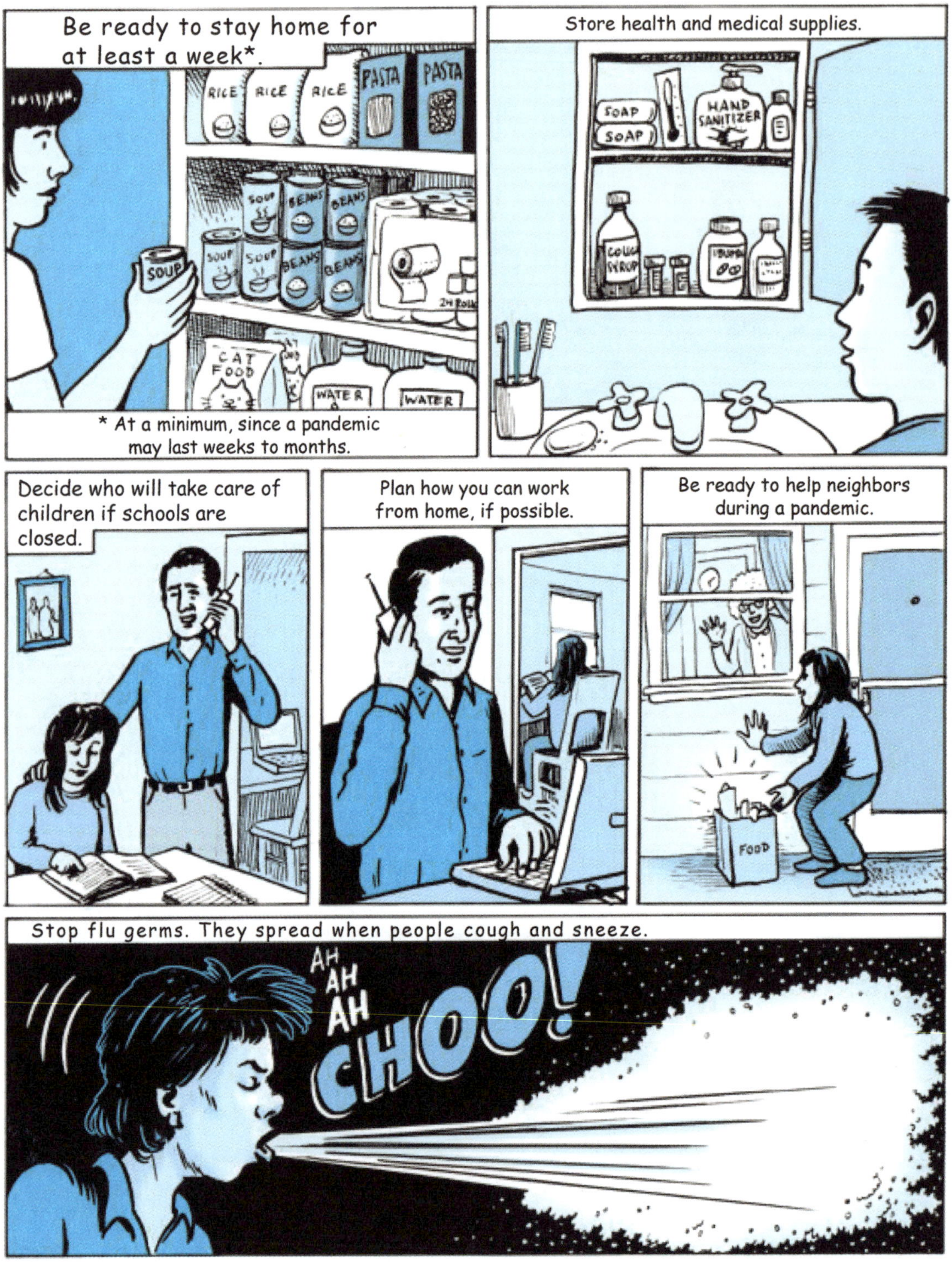
Be ready to stay home for at least a week*.
RICE
RICE
RICE
PASTA
PASTA
SOUP
BEANS
BEANS
SOUP
SOUP
BEANS
BEANS
SOUP
CAT FOOD
WATER
WATER
* At a minimum, since a pandemic may last weeks to months.
Store health and medical supplies.
SOAP
SOAP
HAND SANITIZER
COUGH SYRUP
Decide who will take care of children if schools are closed.
Plan how you can work from home, if possible.
Be ready to help neighbors during a pandemic.
FOOD
Stop flu germs. They spread when people cough and sneeze.
AH
AH
AH
CHOO!

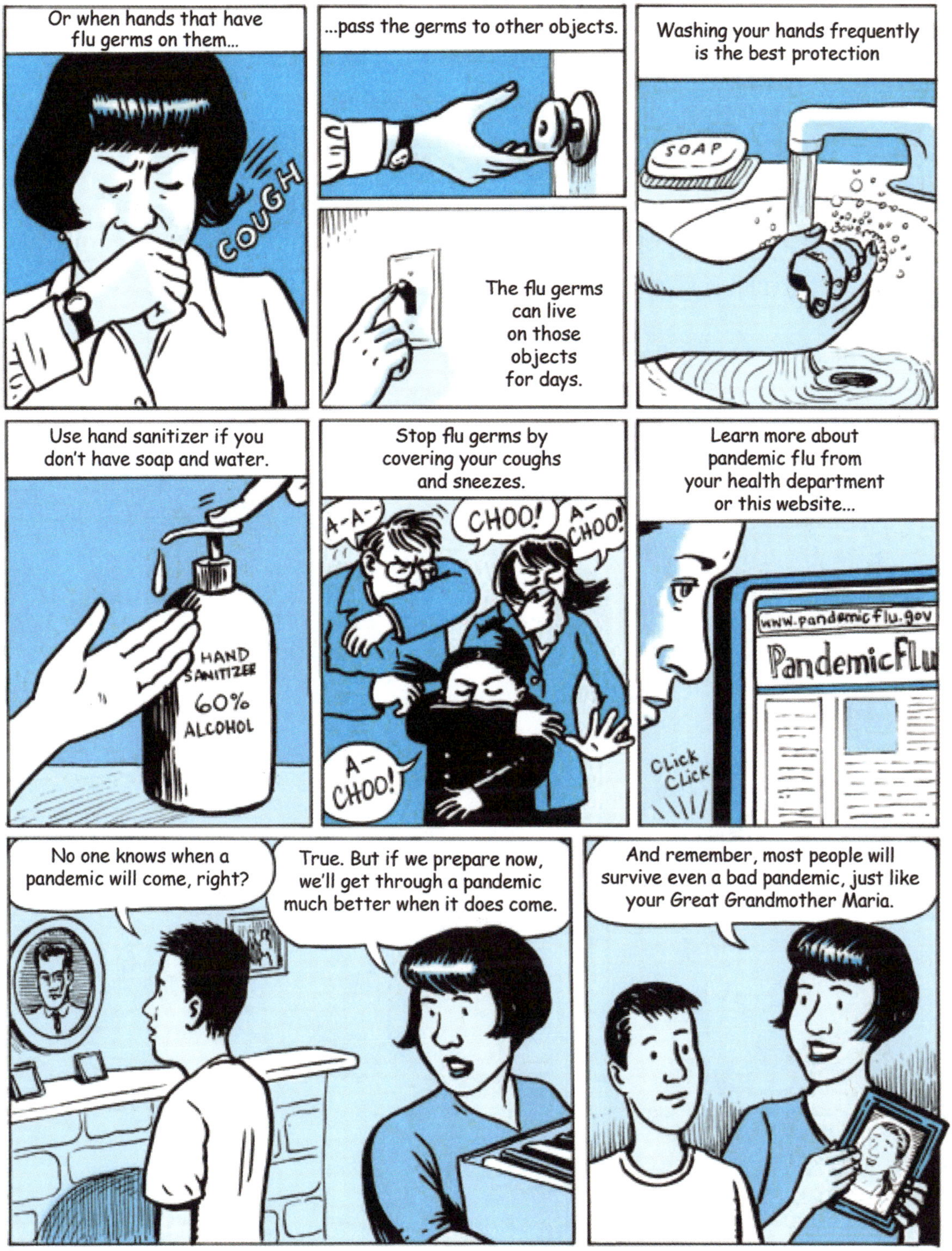
Or when hands that have flu germs on them...
COUGH
...pass the germs to other objects.
The flu germs can live on those objects for days.
Washing your hands frequently is the best protection
SOAP
Use hand sanitizer if you don't have soap and water.
HAND SANITIZER 60% ALCOHOL
Stop flu germs by covering your coughs and sneezes.
A-A--
CHOO!
A-CHOO!
A-CHOO!
Learn more about pandemic flu from your health department or this website...
www.pandemicflu.gov
PandemicFlu
CLick CLick
No one knows when a pandemic will come, right?
True. But if we prepare now, we'll get through a pandemic much better when it does come.
And remember, most people will survive even a bad pandemic, just like your Great Grandmother Maria.

PANDEMIC IN SEATTLE

PART TWO: Seattle Faces a Pandemic

We rejoin a story told by a current Seattleite about her grandparents during the Great Influenza Pandemic...

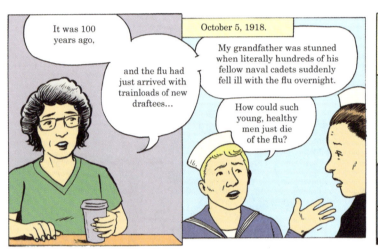

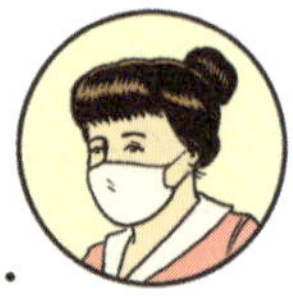

It was 100 years ago,

and the flu had just arrived with trainloads of new draftees...

October 5, 1918.

My grandfather was stunned when literally hundreds of his fellow naval cadets suddenly fell ill with the flu overnight.

How could such young, healthy men just die of the flu?

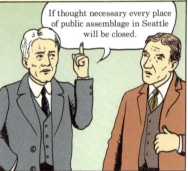

The next day, Seattle's health commissioner, Dr. J.S. McBride, met with Mayor Ole Hanson. Fearing the worst, the mayor supported Health orders to prevent the spread of the flu.

If thought necessary every place of public assemblage in Seattle will be closed.

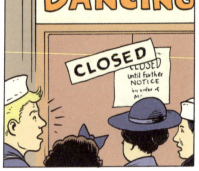

Dance halls, movie theaters, sporting events, church services, "and all entertainments where crowds congregate" were closed and cancelled overnight.

DANCING

CLOSED
until further NOTICE
by order of M-

Seattle public schools and the UW were closed for six weeks, by order of the health department.

!

It will be a relief when school starts again!

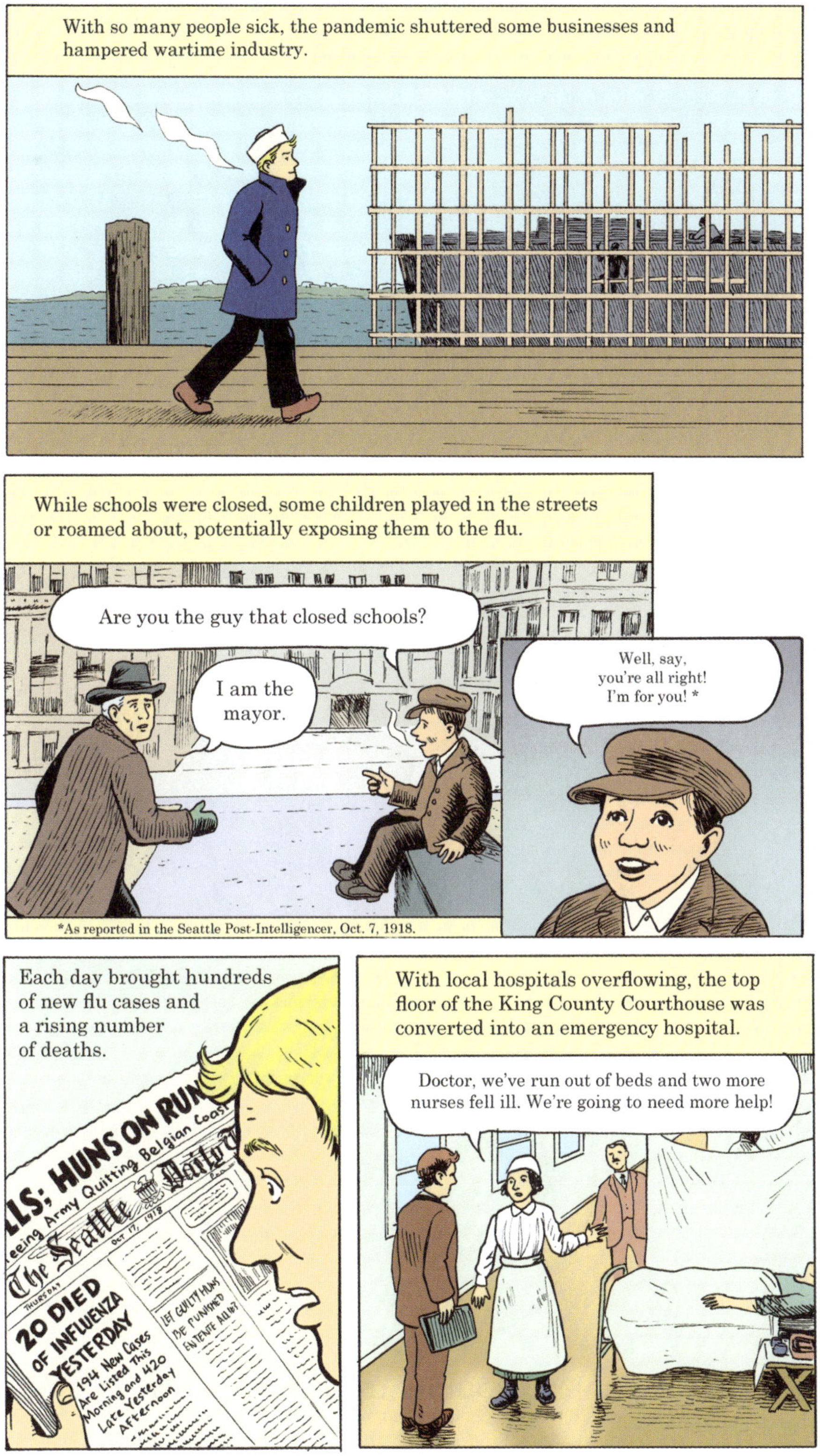

With so many people sick, the pandemic shuttered some businesses and hampered wartime industry.
While schools were closed, some children played in the streets or roamed about, potentially exposing them to the flu.
Are you the guy that closed schools?
I am the mayor.
Well, say, you're all right! I'm for you! *
*As reported in the Seattle Post-Intelligencer, Oct. 7, 1918.
Each day brought hundreds of new flu cases and a rising number of deaths.
The Seattle Daily
20 DIED OF INFLUENZA YESTERDAY
194 New Cases Are Listed This Morning and 420 Late Yesterday Afternoon
LET GUILTY HUNS BE PUNISHED
With local hospitals overflowing, the top floor of the King County Courthouse was converted into an emergency hospital.
Doctor, we've run out of beds and two more nurses fell ill. We're going to need more help!

By the end of the month, flu was so widespread that Dr. McBride issued several controversial measures to try to stop germs in crowded spaces.

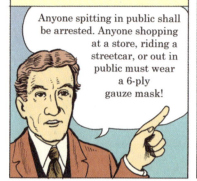

Anyone spitting in public shall be arrested. Anyone shopping at a store, riding a streetcar, or out in public must wear a 6-ply gauze mask!

The masks were hot and uncomfortable. Unfortunately, they probably were little help in filtering out flu viruses.

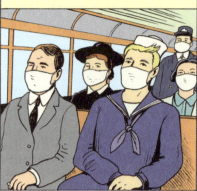

But at the time, people were desperate for some kind of protection. The Red Cross issued a call for volunteers to help make tens of thousands of the "influenza protectors."

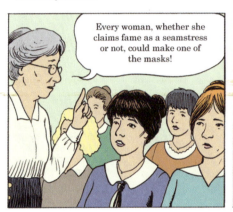

Every woman, whether she claims fame as a seamstress or not, could make one of the masks!

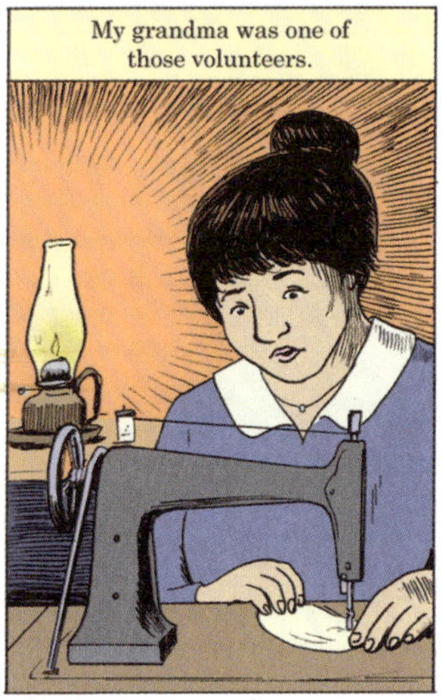

My grandma was one of those volunteers.

Indirectly, the pandemic brought my grandparents together.

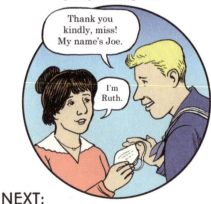

Thank you kindly, miss! My name's Joe.

I'm Ruth.

NEXT:
A city mourns and moves on.

TO BE CONTINUED...

Consult with your doctor on the phone if you are sick

If you are unsure of how to care for yourself or are concerned about your condition, call your health care provider for advice.

Uh-oh
cough cough
RUFF RUFF
Do I feel hot?
Is my throat sore?
I think I'll call my doctor instead of worrying!

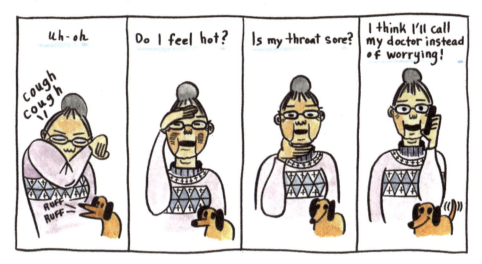

Prevent the spread of COVID-19 in the household

Tips for cleaning and laundry

Clean surfaces that you frequently touch every day with soap and water or other standard cleaning products. This includes countertops, door knobs, handles, and buttons on TV remotes and sink faucets. After scrubbing surfaces clean use a disinfecting cleaner like bleach wipes, bleach spray or other disinfectant spray.

If you cannot find disinfecting cleaner, use a paper towel dipped in rubbing alcohol. The alcohol will kill the virus.

409

Tea

Wash laundry thoroughly using the warmest temperature possible.

Keep the dirty laundry away from your body.

Wash your hands immediately after handling laundry.

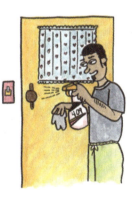

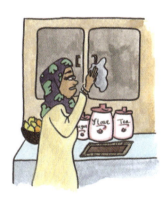

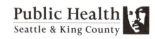

Public Health
Seattle & King County

Living in a multigenerational household

When there are multiple people in the household, there can be additional risk for older relatives who are more vulnerable to serious illness from COVID-19.

If you have older adults living at home, or family members with medical conditions, take the following steps to protect them from possible infection:

If you have to go outside the home

Take these steps to protect yourself and prevent carrying the virus into your home:

- Wear a cloth mask which covers your mouth and nose.
- Stay at least 6 feet away from others.
- Carry hand sanitizer or disinfecting wipes with you so that you can disinfect surfaces before you touch them or sanitize your hands.
- Travel alone, if possible. Try not to bring children with you. They are more likely to touch things in public and could carry those germs back to your home.

If you are an essential worker

Before leaving work, wash your hands with soap and water for at least 20 seconds. When returning home from work, change your clothes and shoes and wash your hands, especially if you've had any interaction with others. Children who go to childcare should take the same steps.

Let's change clothes and clean up for grandma!

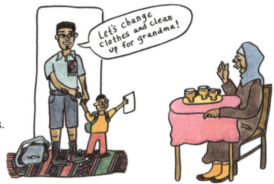

Inside the home

If you are exposed to coronavirus, you might not know it. So even inside your home, it is important to maintain social distancing as best you can. If possible, spend time in separate rooms from vulnerable family members. If you cannot separate, try to stay 6 feet away from vulnerable family members when in the same room.

I drew an apple for you grandma!

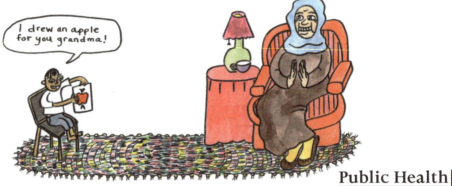

Public Health
Seattle & King County

Providing care

If you are the primary caregiver for an older adult in your home, and you help them with daily activities like bathing and getting dressed, take extra precaution by:

- Wash your hands thoroughly before providing care.
- Wear a cloth face covering when providing care. Cloth face coverings should be worn by you and the person receiving care.
- If you use towels and wash cloths, make sure to use clean ones each time.

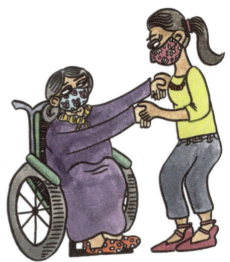

Preparing and sharing meals

- Wash your hands before, during, and after preparing food.
- Wash utensils and surfaces after each use.
- Cook foods to a high enough temperature to kill germs that can make you sick or give you food poisoning.
- During meals, try to maintain 6 feet of distance between family members.
- If prayer is part of your family's mealtime routine, pray without holding hands.

Practice healthy habits

I wanna show grandma my drawing!
After we wash!

Every family member should practice healthy habits so they don't get sick and expose vulnerable members of the household.

- Wash hands frequently with soap and water for at least 20 seconds.
- Avoid touching your eyes, nose, or mouth with unwashed hands.
- Cover coughs and sneezes with a tissue or a sleeve.

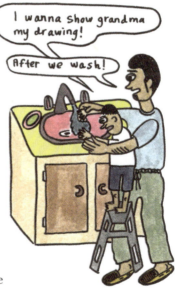

Enjoy Time Together

Despite the challenges of this outbreak, living with older family members has so many benefits, including keeping strong bonds across generations. Finding safe ways to continue to interact and demonstrate your affection for one another is important.

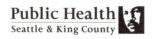

Public Health
Seattle & King County

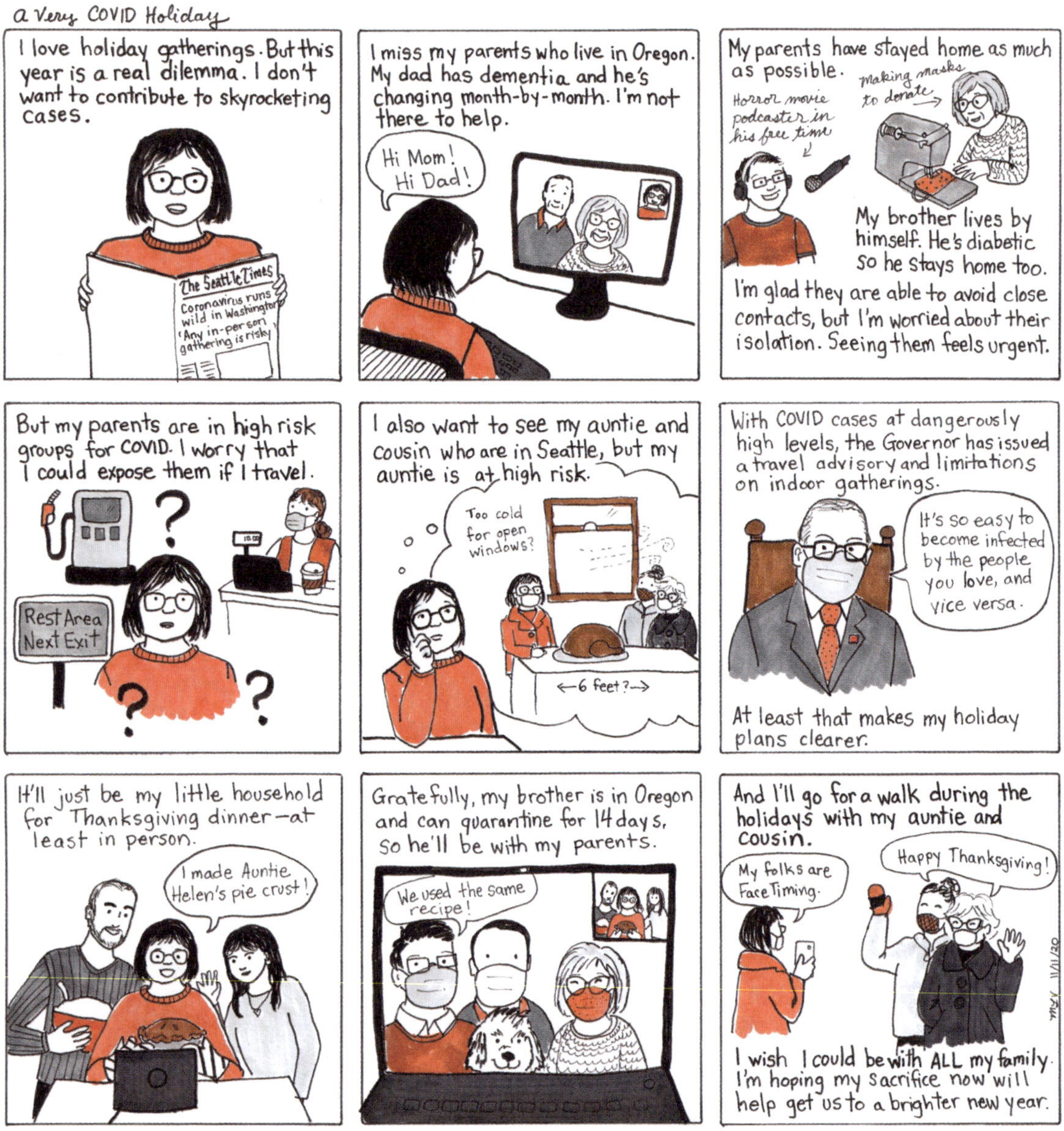
a Very COVID Holiday
I love holiday gatherings. But this year is a real dilemma. I don't want to contribute to skyrocketing cases.
The Seattle Times
Coronavirus runs wild in Washington
'Any in-person gathering is risky'
I miss my parents who live in Oregon. My dad has dementia and he's changing month-by-month. I'm not there to help.
Hi Mom! Hi Dad!
My parents have stayed home as much as possible.
Horror movie podcaster in his free time
Making masks to donate
My brother lives by himself. He's diabetic so he stays home too.
I'm glad they are able to avoid close contacts, but I'm worried about their isolation. Seeing them feels urgent.
But my parents are in high risk groups for COVID. I worry that I could expose them if I travel.
Rest Area Next Exit
I also want to see my auntie and cousin who are in Seattle, but my auntie is at high risk.
Too cold for open windows?
←6 feet?→
With COVID cases at dangerously high levels, the Governor has issued a travel advisory and limitations on indoor gatherings.
It's so easy to become infected by the people you love, and vice versa.
At least that makes my holiday plans clearer.
It'll just be my little household for Thanksgiving dinner—at least in person.
I made Auntie Helen's pie crust!
Gratefully, my brother is in Oregon and can quarantine for 14 days, so he'll be with my parents.
We used the same recipe!
And I'll go for a walk during the holidays with my auntie and cousin.
My folks are FaceTiming.
Happy Thanksgiving!
11/11/20
I wish I could be with ALL my family. I'm hoping my sacrifice now will help get us to a brighter new year.

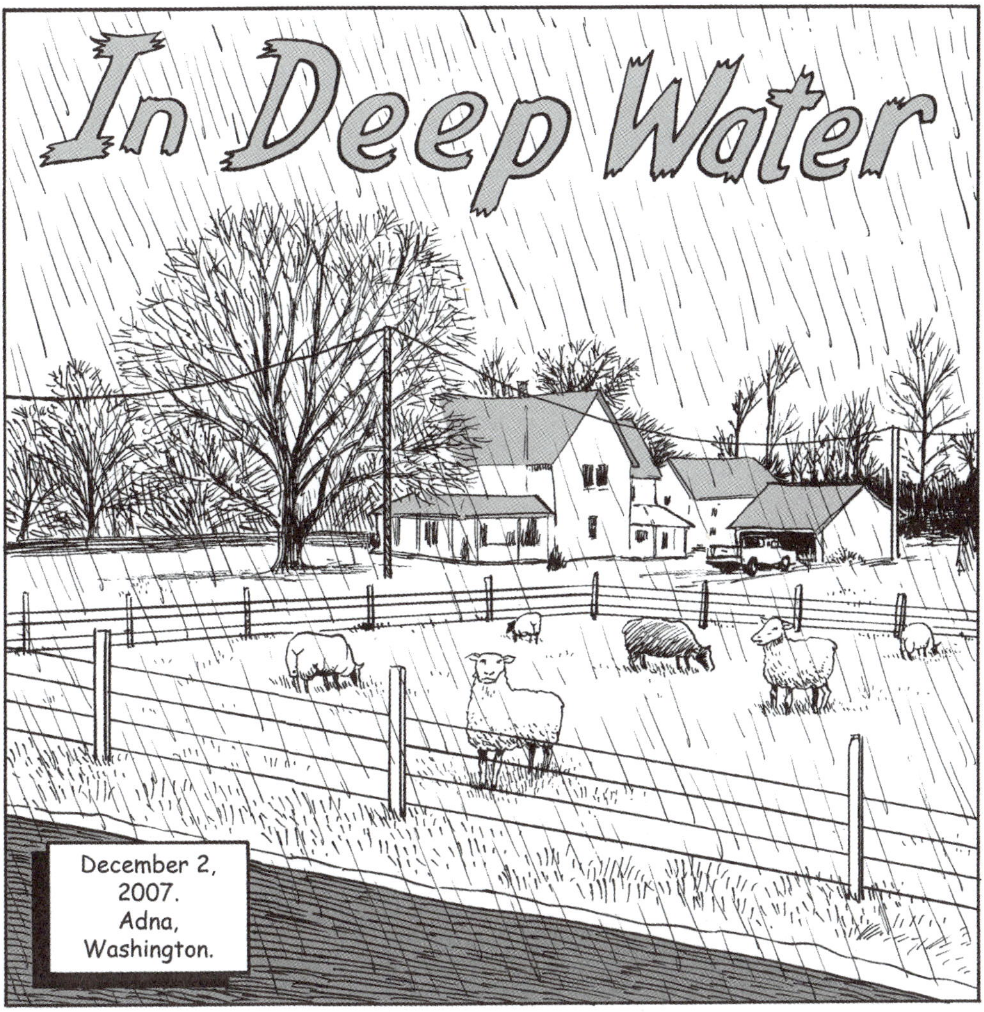
In Deep Water
December 2, 2007. Adna, Washington.

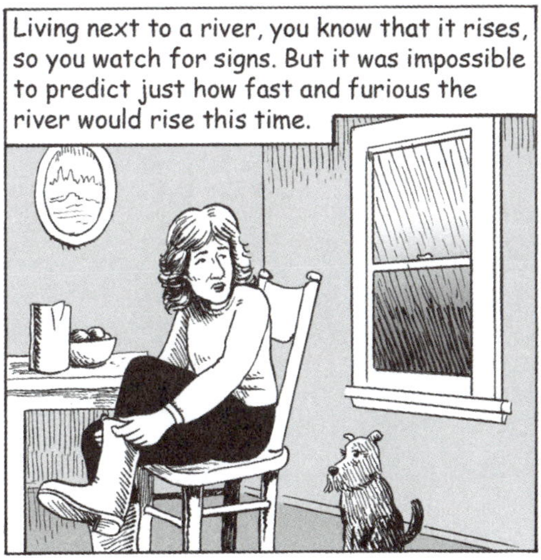
Living next to a river, you know that it rises, so you watch for signs. But it was impossible to predict just how fast and furious the river would rise this time.

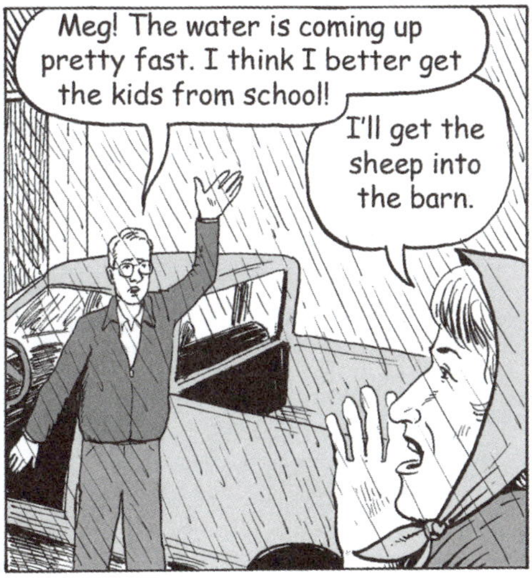
Meg! The water is coming up pretty fast. I think I better get the kids from school!
I'll get the sheep into the barn.

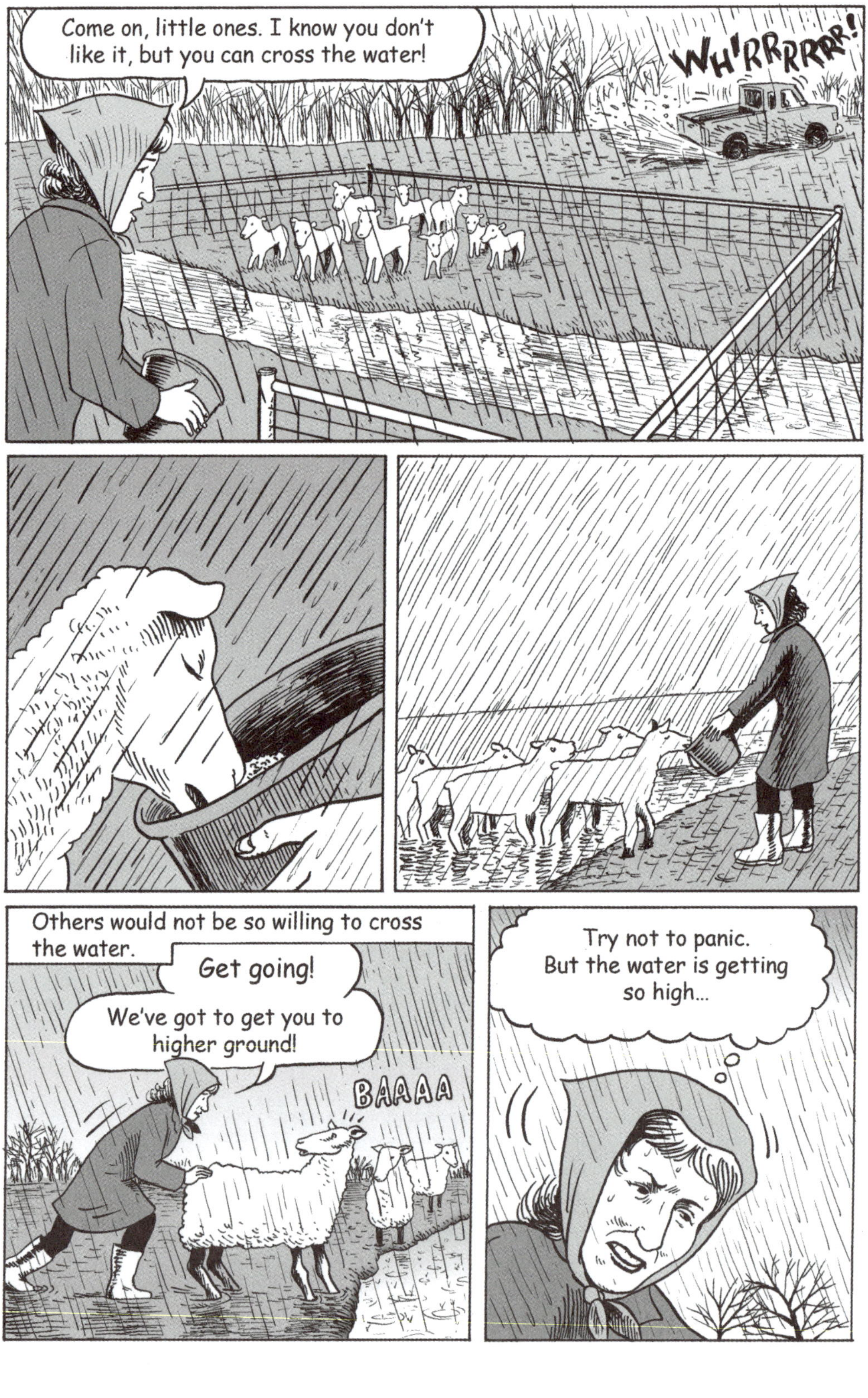
Come on, little ones. I know you don't like it, but you can cross the water!
WH'RRRRRR!
Others would not be so willing to cross the water.
Get going!
We've got to get you to higher ground!
BAAAA
Try not to panic. But the water is getting so high...

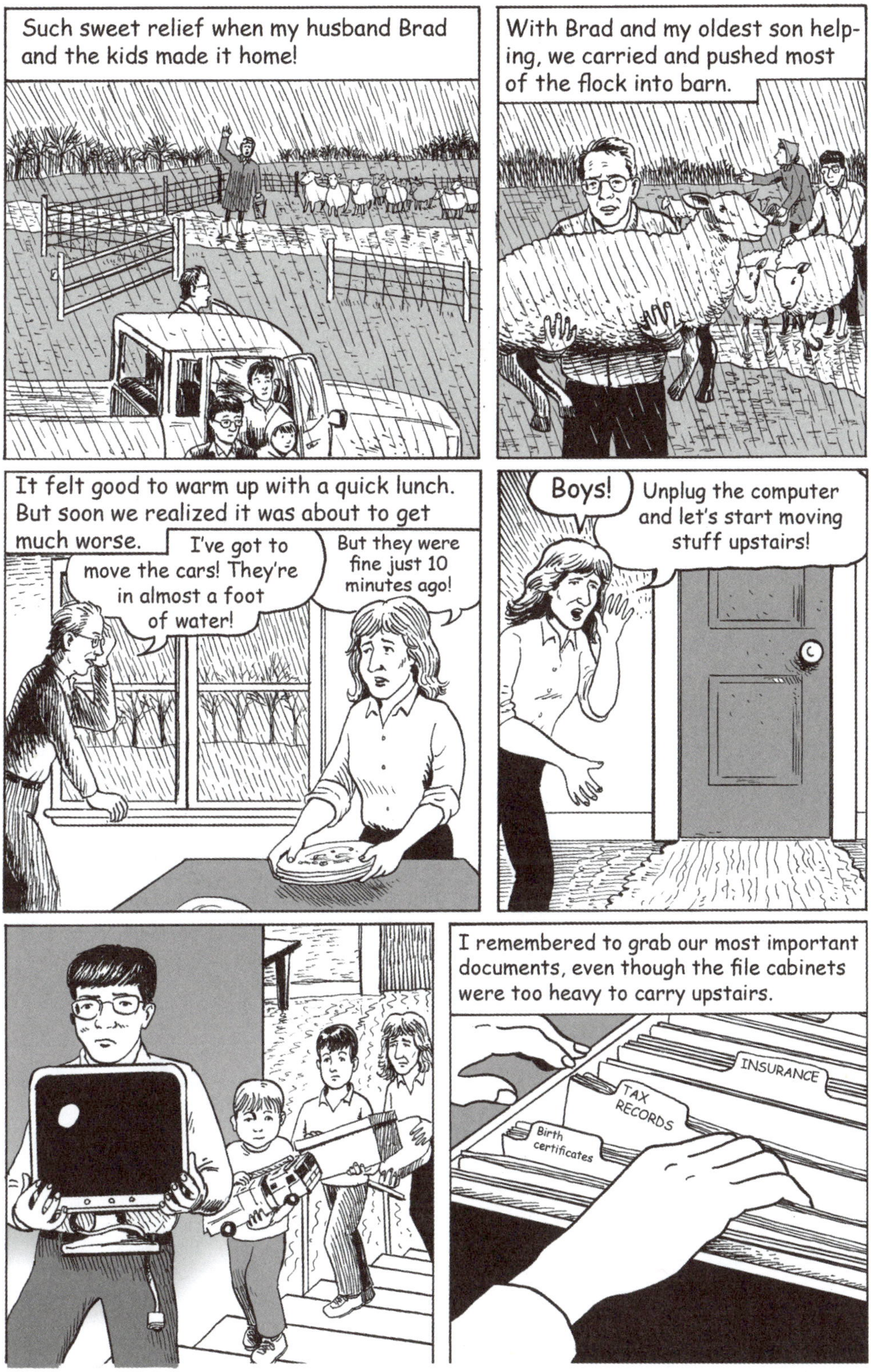
Such sweet relief when my husband Brad and the kids made it home!
With Brad and my oldest son help-ing, we carried and pushed most of the flock into barn.
It felt good to warm up with a quick lunch. But soon we realized it was about to get much worse.
I've got to move the cars! They're in almost a foot of water!
But they were fine just 10 minutes ago!
Boys!
Unplug the computer and let's start moving stuff upstairs!
I remembered to grab our most important documents, even though the file cabinets were too heavy to carry upstairs.
INSURANCE
TAX RECORDS
Birth certificates

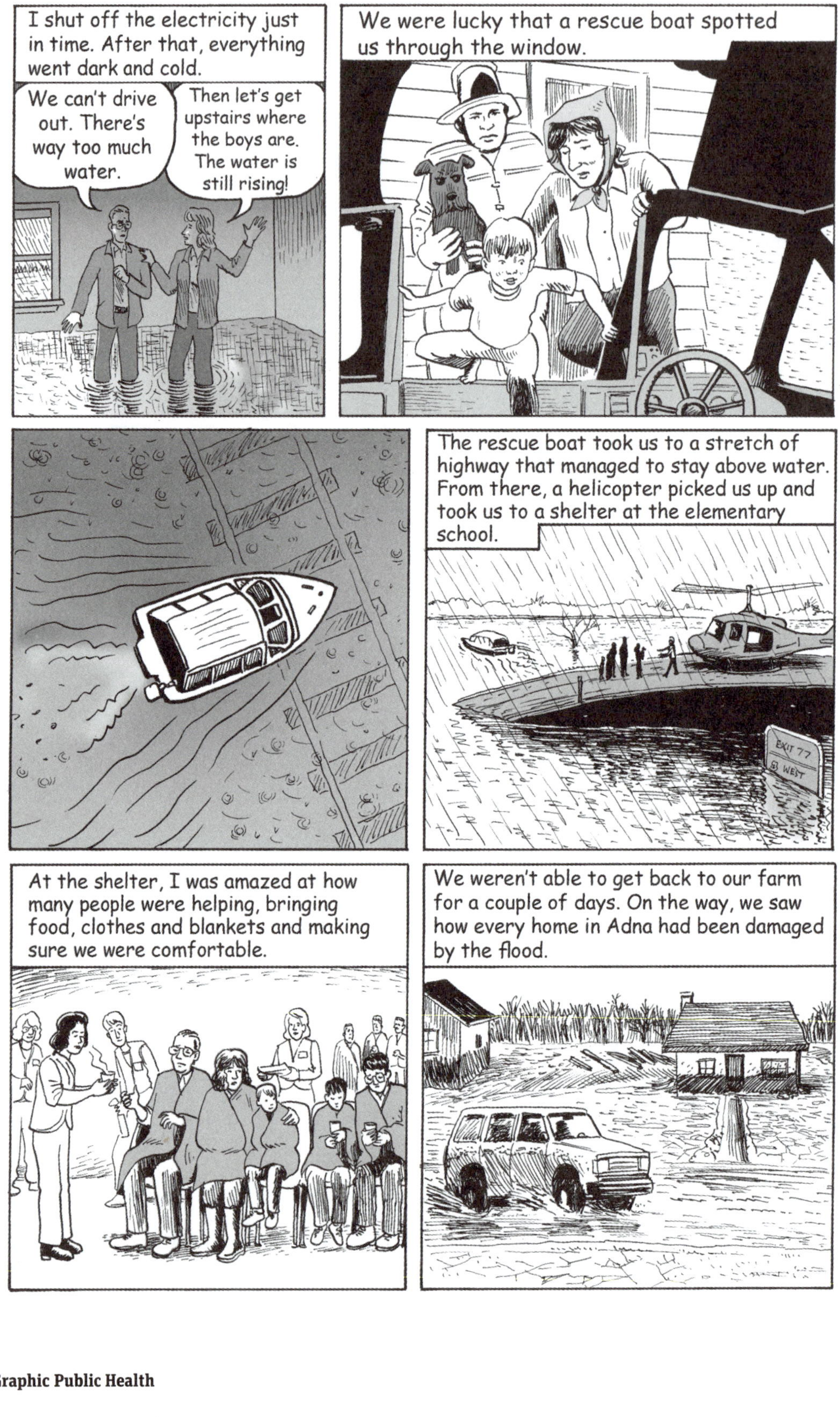
I shut off the electricity just in time. After that, everything went dark and cold.
We can't drive out. There's way too much water.
Then let's get upstairs where the boys are. The water is still rising!
We were lucky that a rescue boat spotted us through the window.
The rescue boat took us to a stretch of highway that managed to stay above water. From there, a helicopter picked us up and took us to a shelter at the elementary school.
EXIT 77
At the shelter, I was amazed at how many people were helping, bringing food, clothes and blankets and making sure we were comfortable.
We weren't able to get back to our farm for a couple of days. On the way, we saw how every home in Adna had been damaged by the flood.

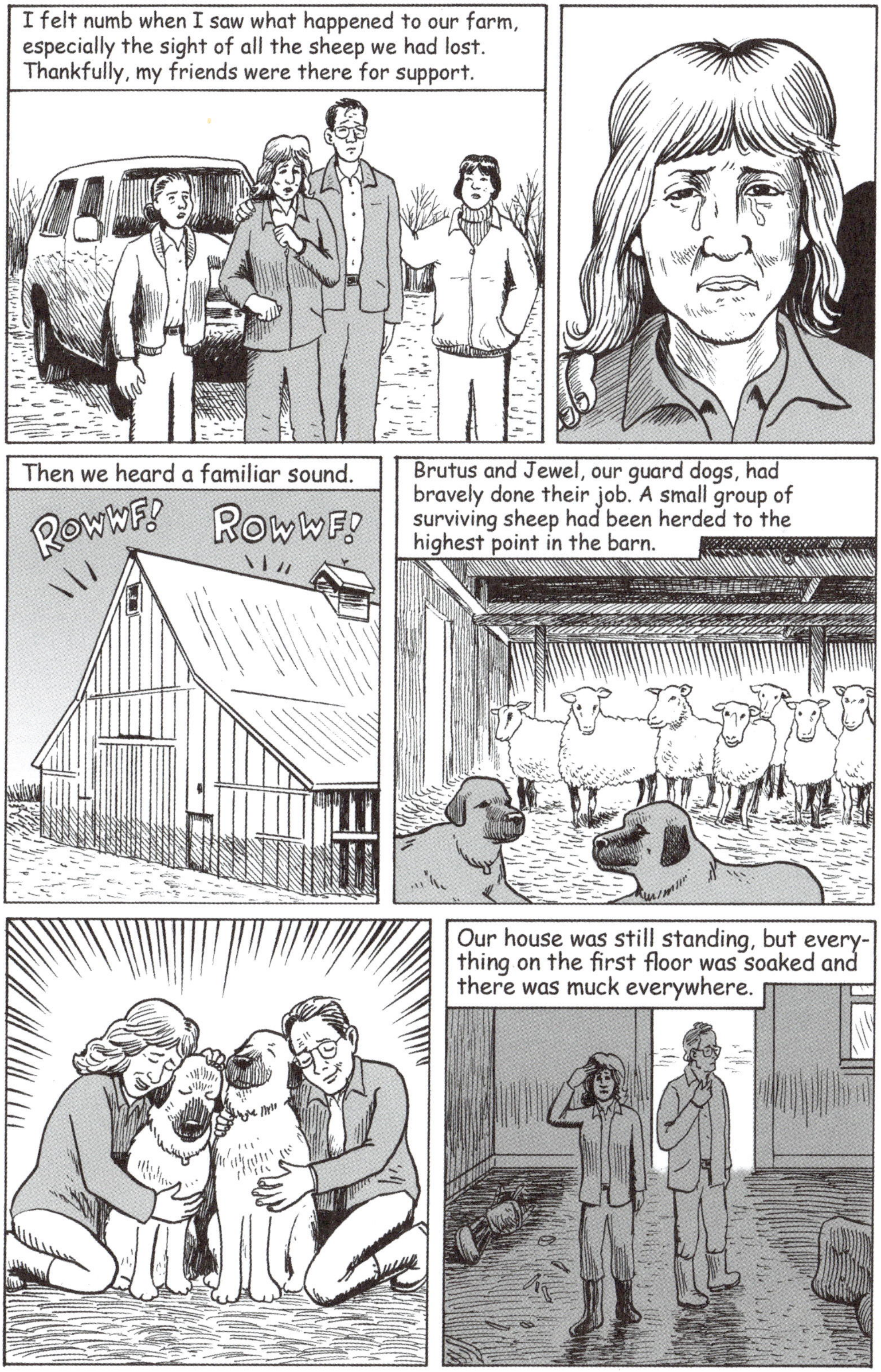
I felt numb when I saw what happened to our farm, especially the sight of all the sheep we had lost. Thankfully, my friends were there for support.
Then we heard a familiar sound.
ROWWF!
ROWWF!
Brutus and Jewel, our guard dogs, had bravely done their job. A small group of surviving sheep had been herded to the highest point in the barn.
Our house was still standing, but every-thing on the first floor was soaked and there was muck everywhere.

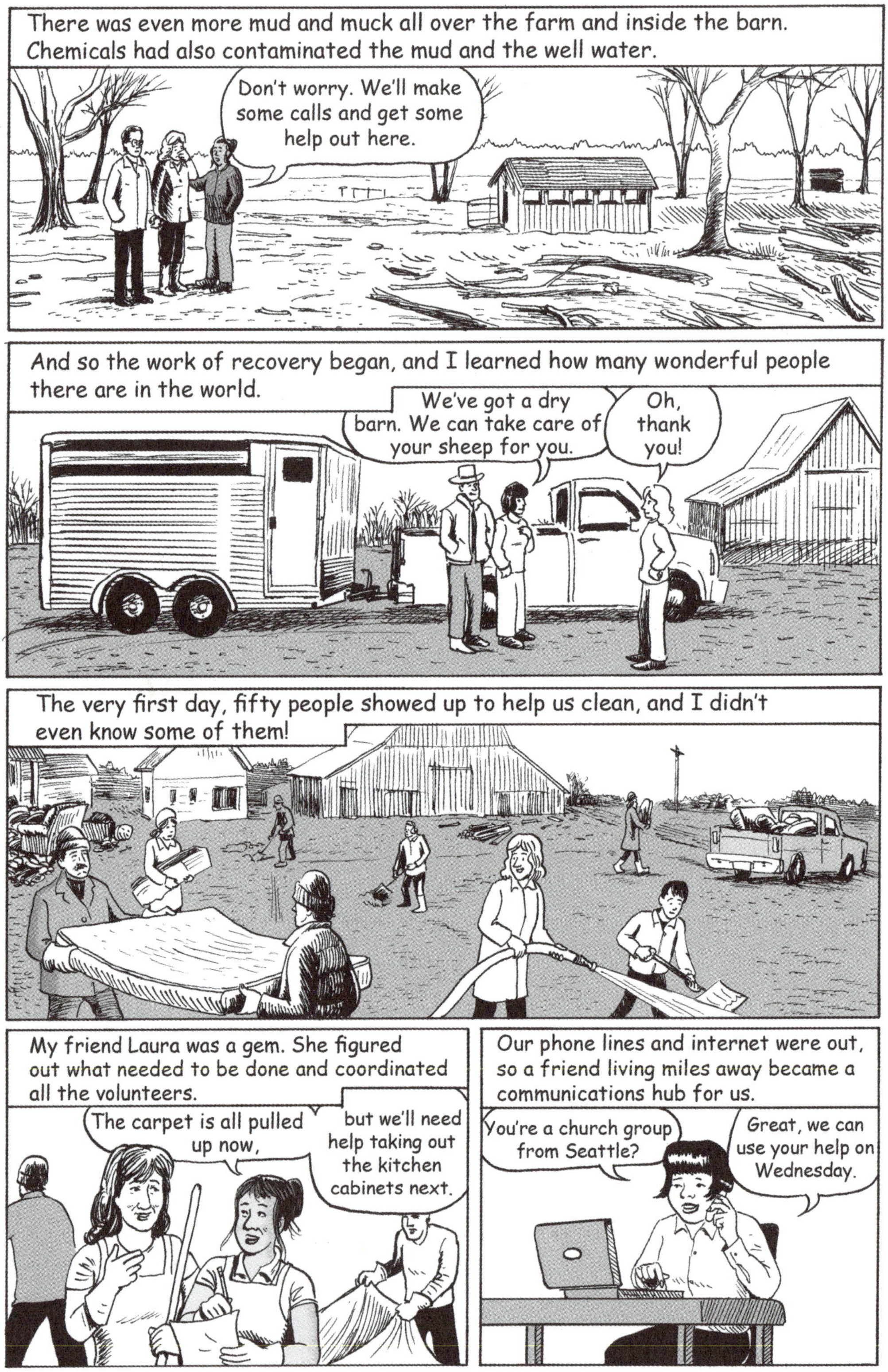
There was even more mud and muck all over the farm and inside the barn. Chemicals had also contaminated the mud and the well water.
Don't worry. We'll make some calls and get some help out here.
And so the work of recovery began, and I learned how many wonderful people there are in the world.
We've got a dry barn. We can take care of your sheep for you.
Oh, thank you!
The very first day, fifty people showed up to help us clean, and I didn't even know some of them!
My friend Laura was a gem. She figured out what needed to be done and coordinated all the volunteers.
The carpet is all pulled up now,
but we'll need help taking out the kitchen cabinets next.
Our phone lines and internet were out, so a friend living miles away became a communications hub for us.
You're a church group from Seattle?
Great, we can use your help on Wednesday.

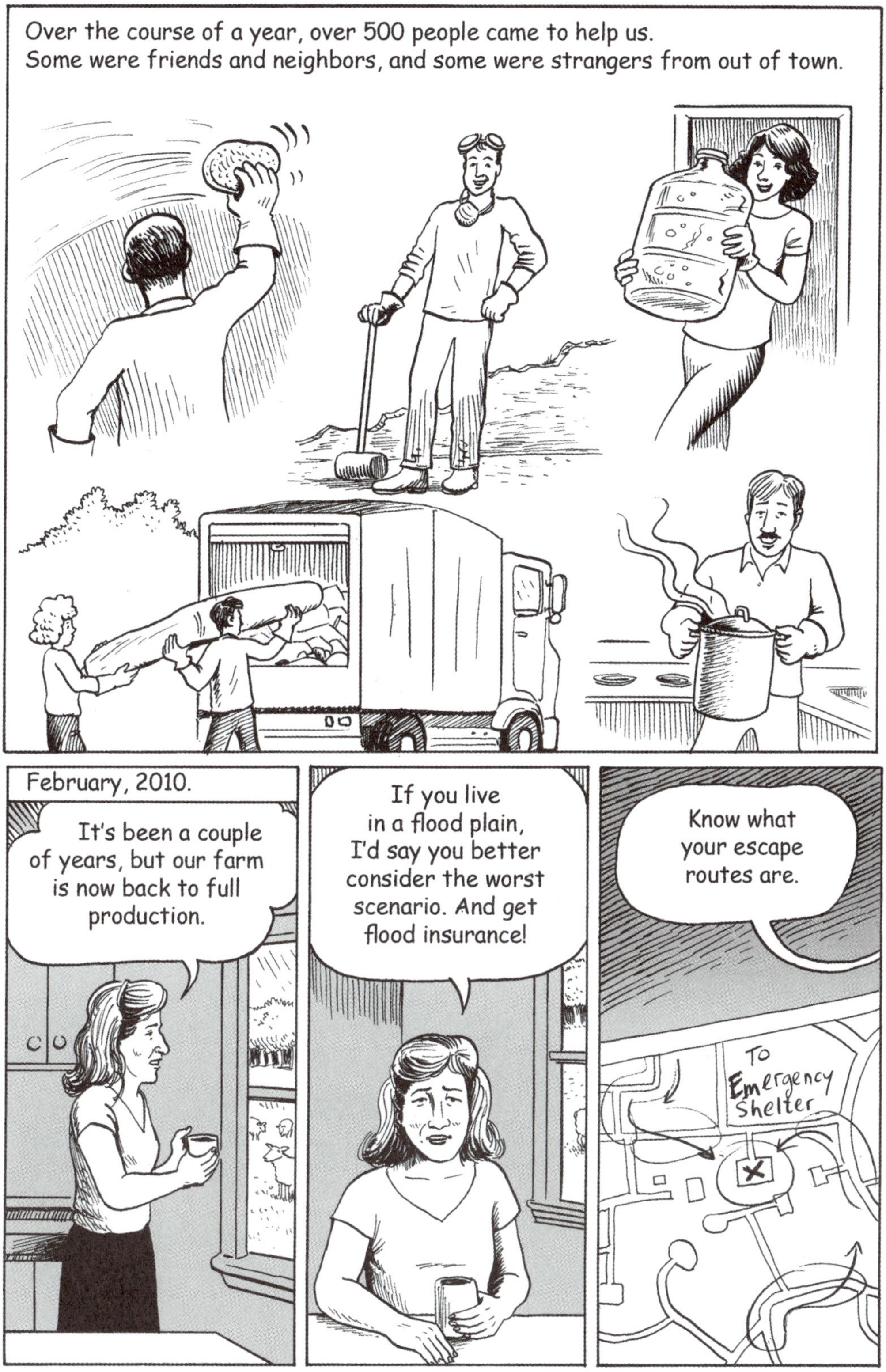
Over the course of a year, over 500 people came to help us.
Some were friends and neighbors, and some were strangers from out of town.
February, 2010.
It's been a couple of years, but our farm is now back to full production.
If you live in a flood plain, I'd say you better consider the worst scenario. And get flood insurance!
Know what your escape routes are.
To Emergency Shelter

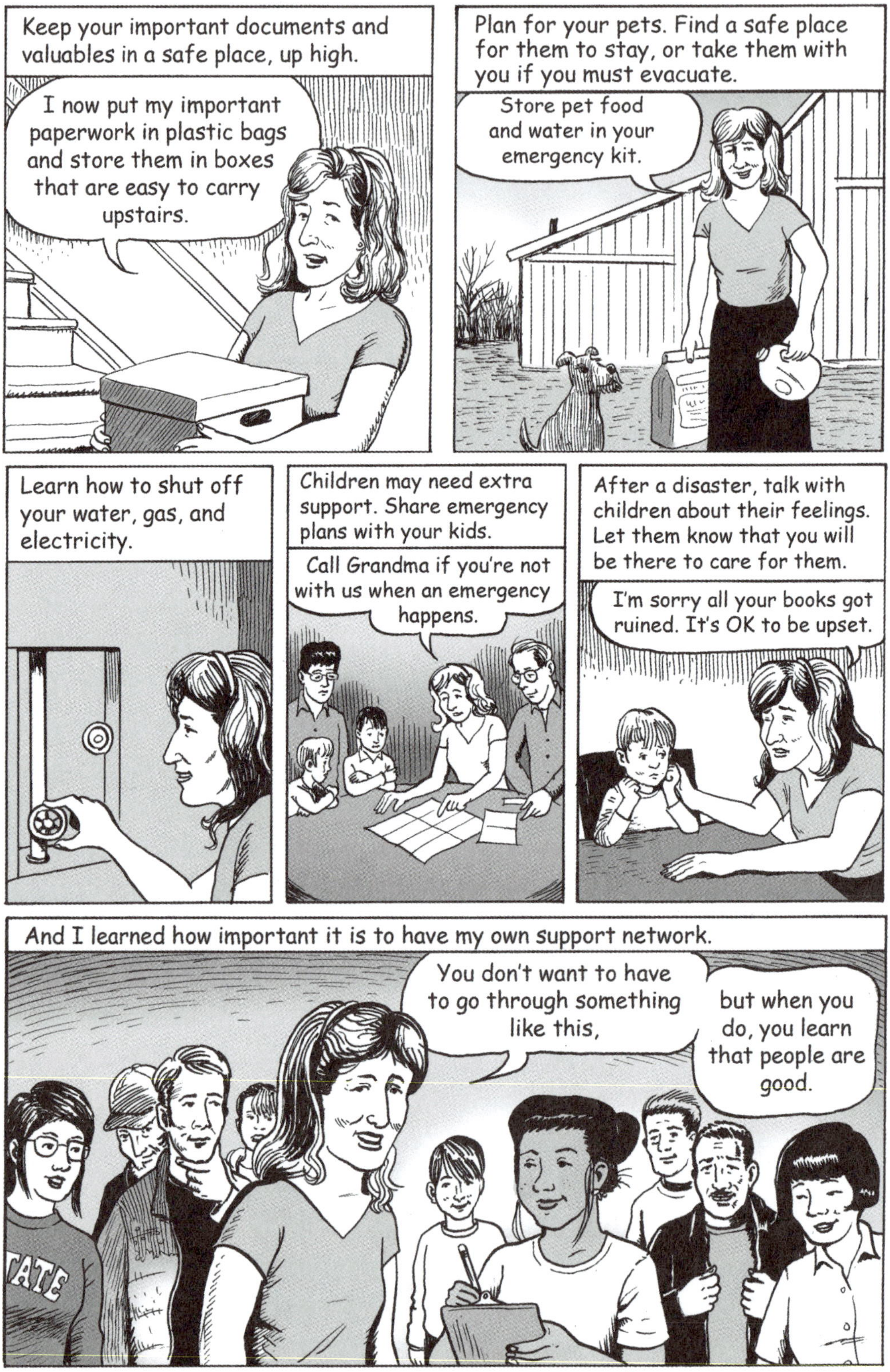
Keep your important documents and valuables in a safe place, up high.
I now put my important paperwork in plastic bags and store them in boxes that are easy to carry upstairs.
Plan for your pets. Find a safe place for them to stay, or take them with you if you must evacuate.
Store pet food and water in your emergency kit.
Learn how to shut off your water, gas, and electricity.
Children may need extra support. Share emergency plans with your kids.
Call Grandma if you're not with us when an emergency happens.
After a disaster, talk with children about their feelings. Let them know that you will be there to care for them.
I'm sorry all your books got ruined. It's OK to be upset.
And I learned how important it is to have my own support network.
You don't want to have to go through something like this,
but when you do, you learn that people are good.
TATE

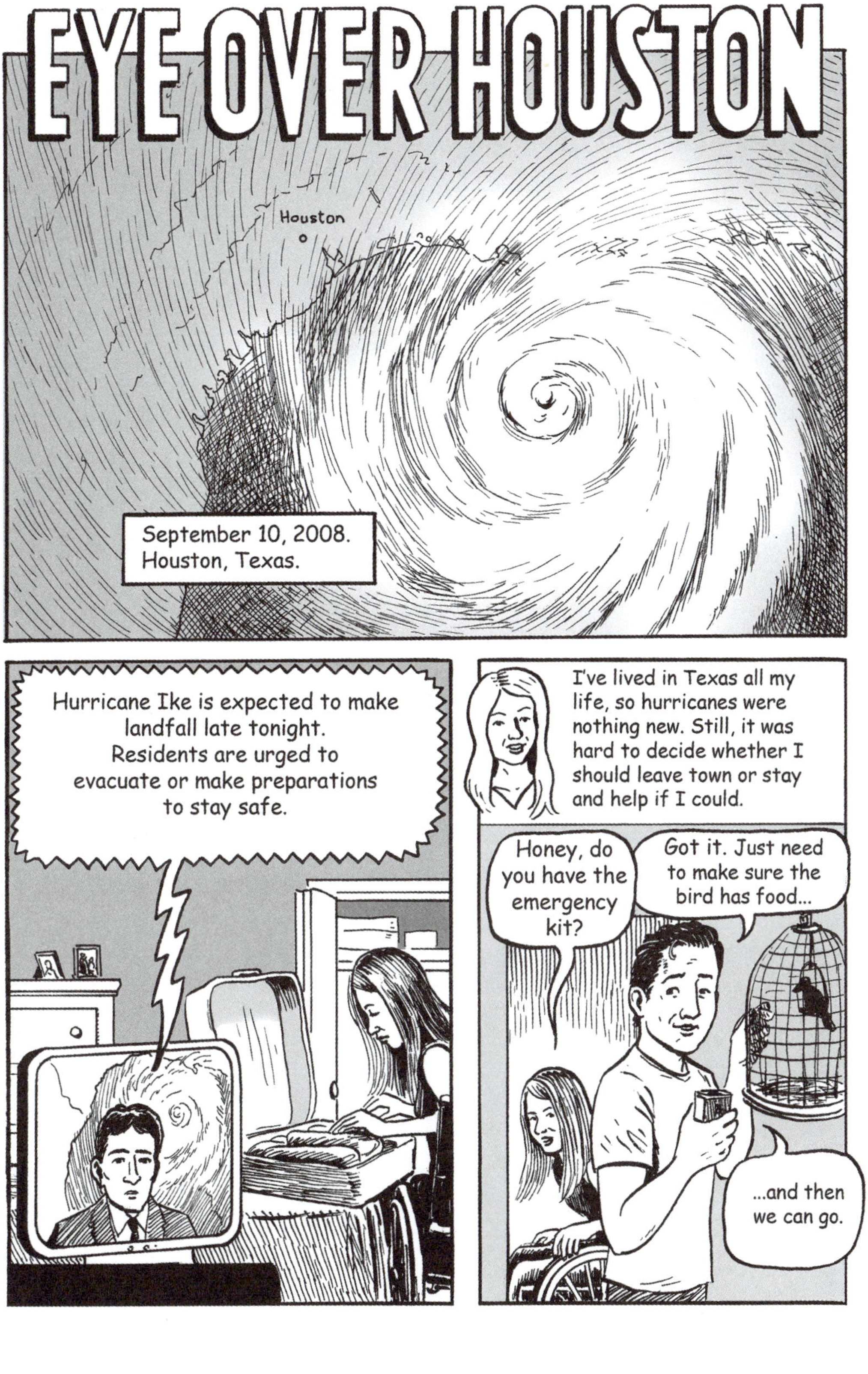
EYE OVER HOUSTON
Houston
September 10, 2008.
Houston, Texas.
Hurricane Ike is expected to make landfall late tonight. Residents are urged to evacuate or make preparations to stay safe.
I've lived in Texas all my life, so hurricanes were nothing new. Still, it was hard to decide whether I should leave town or stay and help if I could.
Honey, do you have the emergency kit?
Got it. Just need to make sure the bird has food...
...and then we can go.

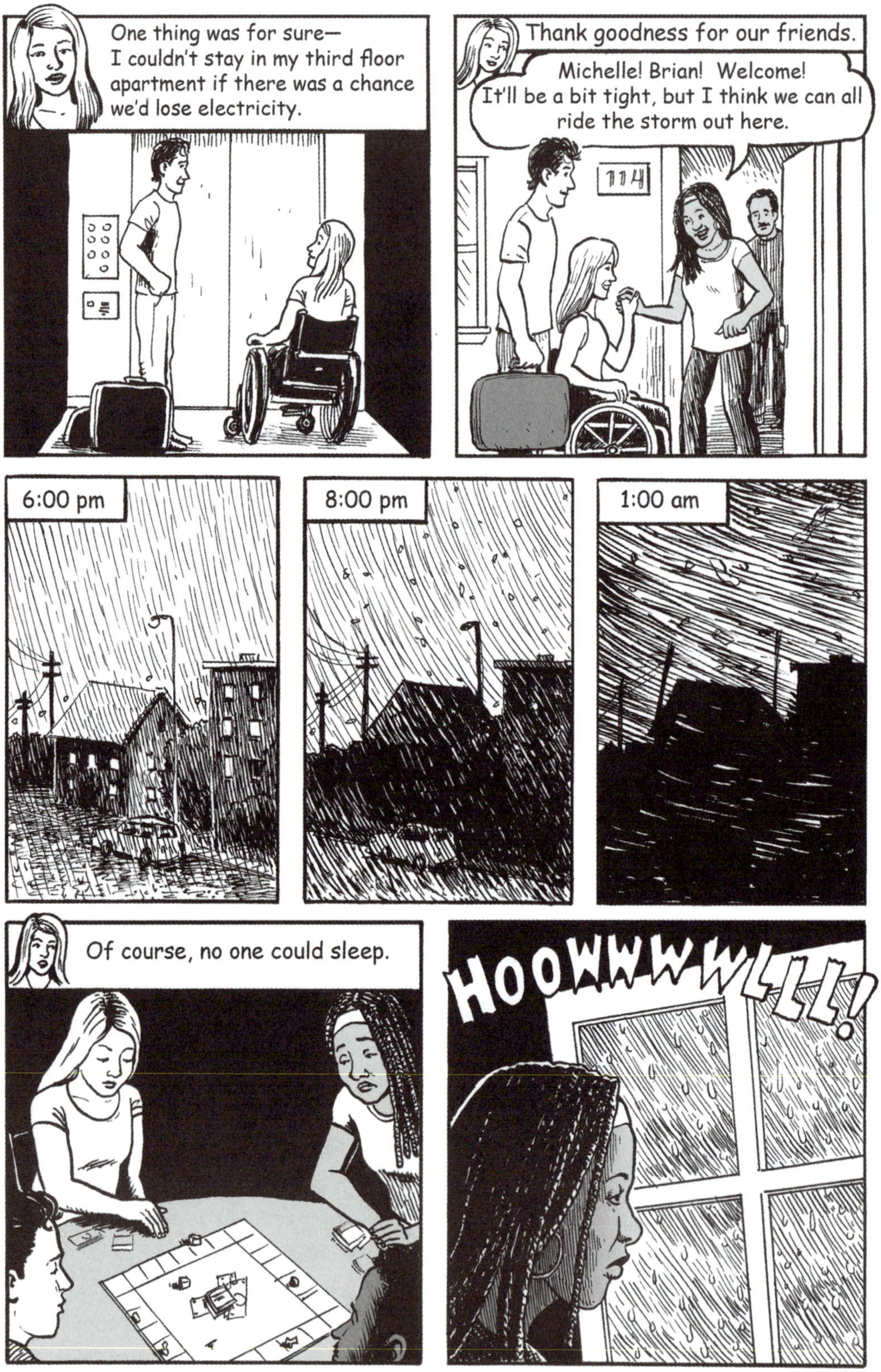
One thing was for sure— I couldn't stay in my third floor apartment if there was a chance we'd lose electricity.
Thank goodness for our friends.
Michelle! Brian! Welcome! It'll be a bit tight, but I think we can all ride the storm out here.
114
6:00 pm
8:00 pm
1:00 am
Of course, no one could sleep.
HOOWWWWLLL!

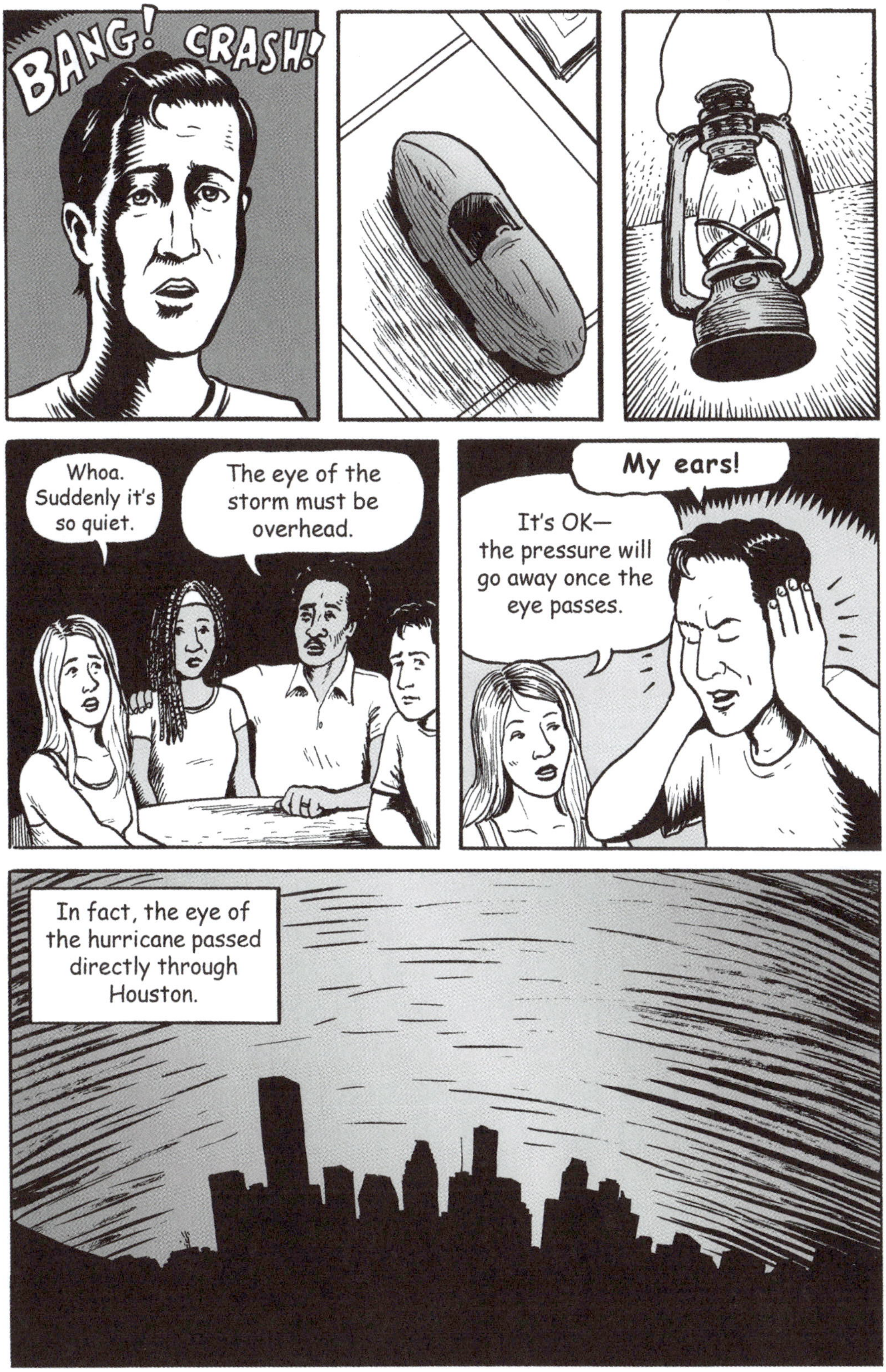
BANG! CRASH!
Whoa. Suddenly it's so quiet.
The eye of the storm must be overhead.
My ears!
It's OK— the pressure will go away once the eye passes.
In fact, the eye of the hurricane passed directly through Houston.

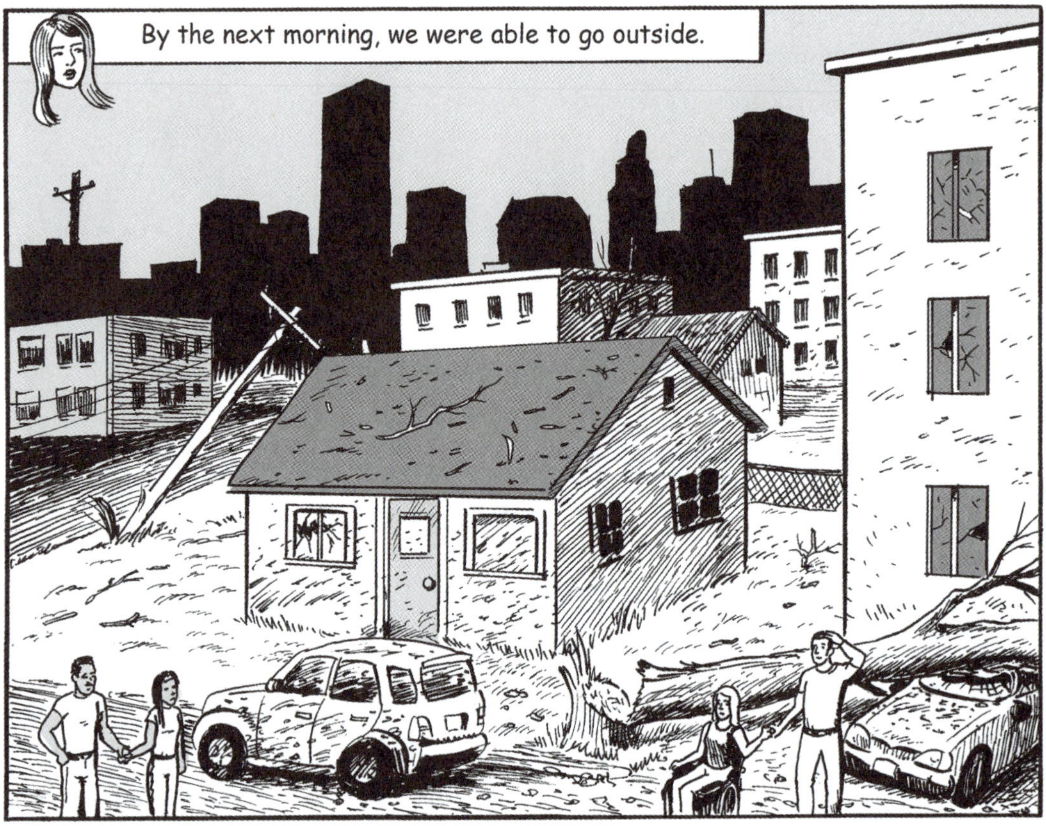
By the next morning, we were able to go outside.

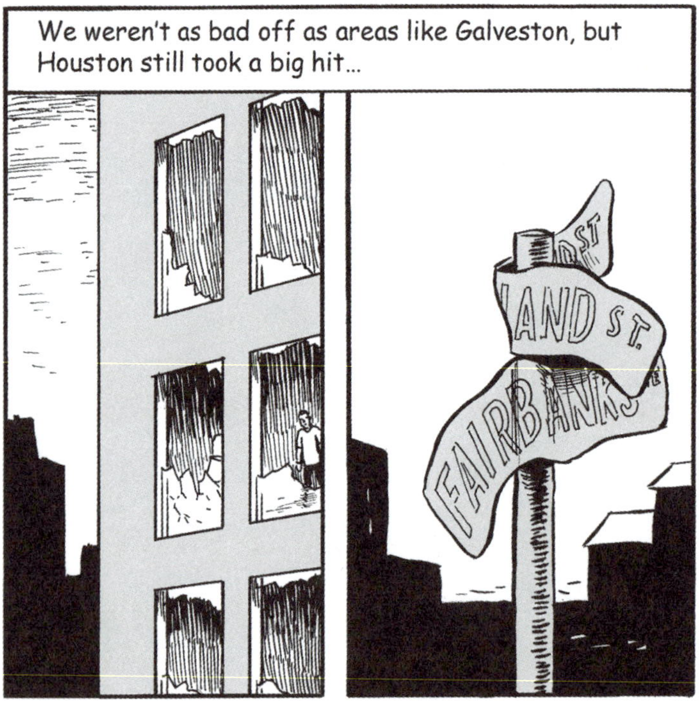
We weren't as bad off as areas like Galveston, but Houston still took a big hit...
LAND ST.
FAIRBANKS

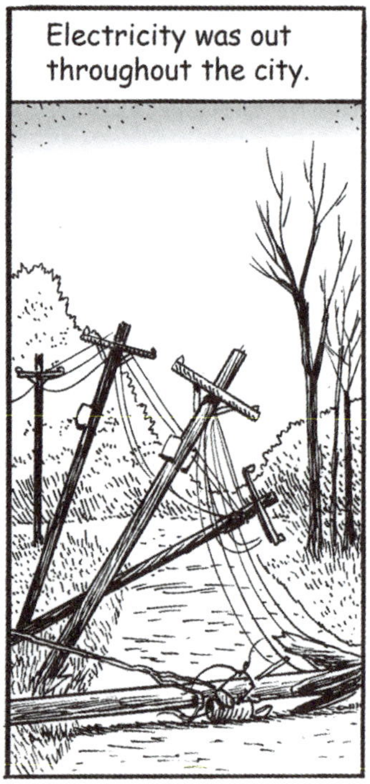
Electricity was out throughout the city.

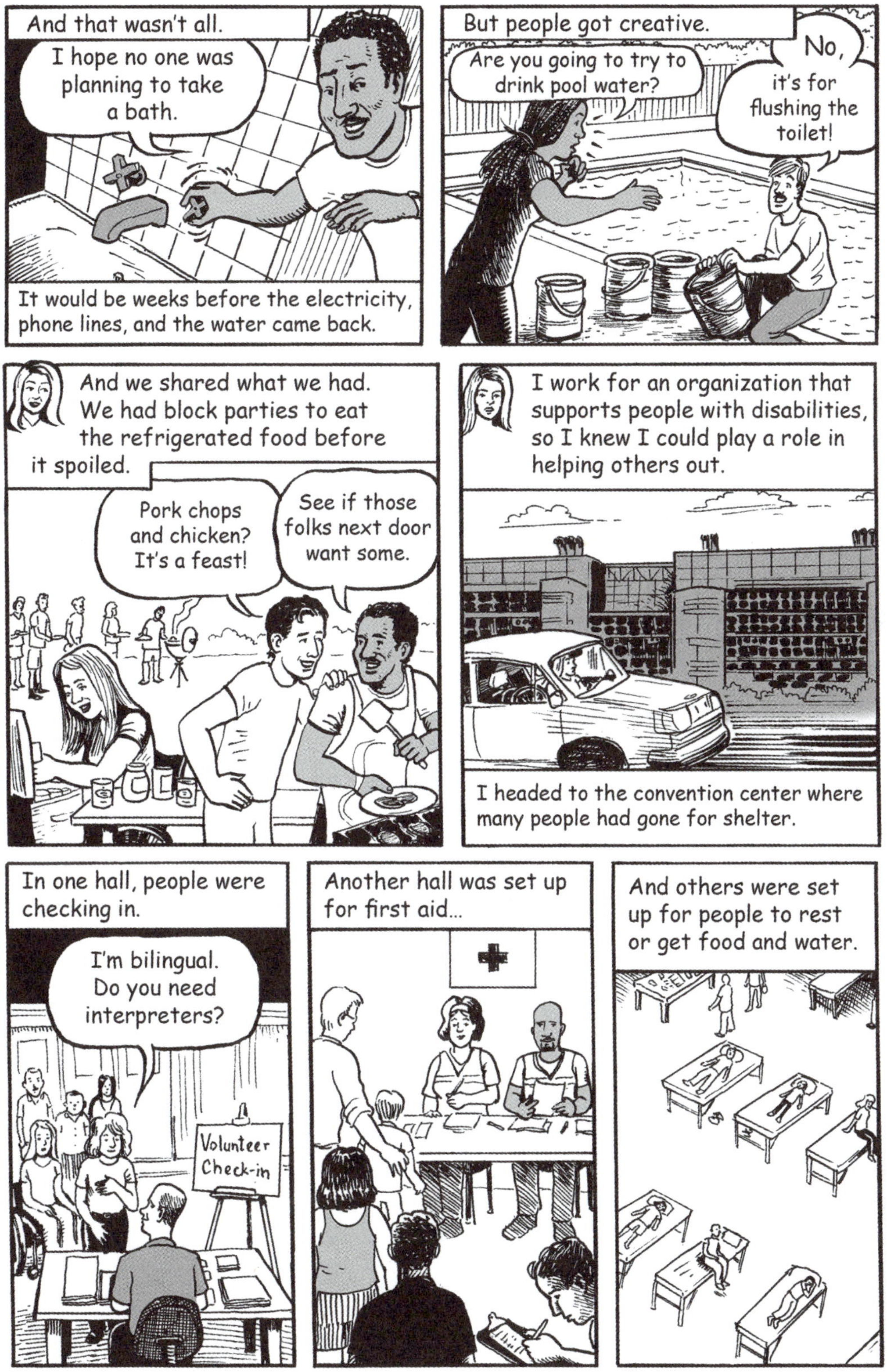
And that wasn't all.
I hope no one was planning to take a bath.
It would be weeks before the electricity, phone lines, and the water came back.
But people got creative.
Are you going to try to drink pool water?
No, it's for flushing the toilet!
And we shared what we had. We had block parties to eat the refrigerated food before it spoiled.
Pork chops and chicken? It's a feast!
See if those folks next door want some.
I work for an organization that supports people with disabilities, so I knew I could play a role in helping others out.
I headed to the convention center where many people had gone for shelter.
In one hall, people were checking in.
I'm bilingual. Do you need interpreters?
Volunteer Check-in
Another hall was set up for first aid...
And others were set up for people to rest or get food and water.

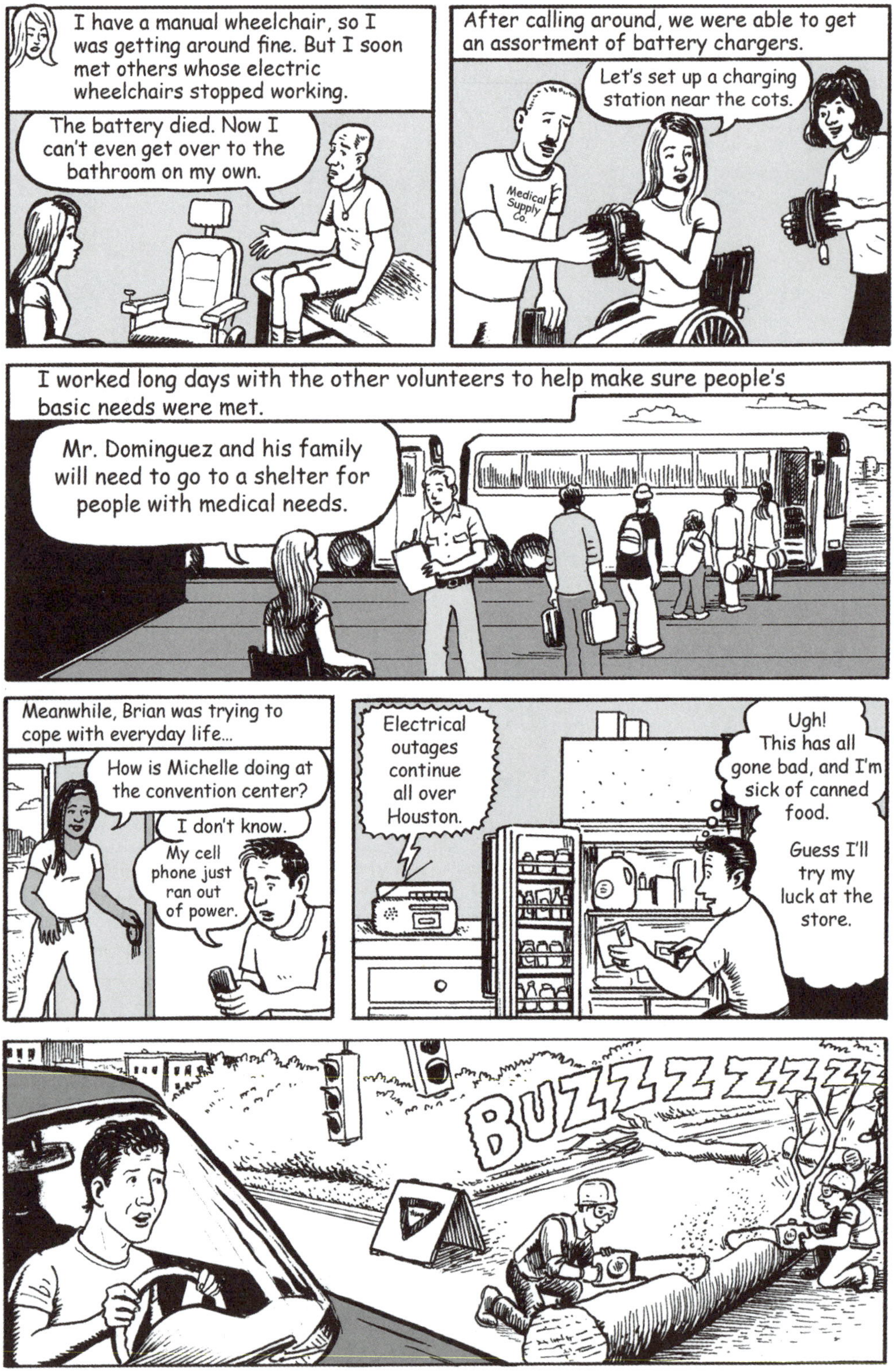
I have a manual wheelchair, so I was getting around fine. But I soon met others whose electric wheelchairs stopped working.
The battery died. Now I can't even get over to the bathroom on my own.
After calling around, we were able to get an assortment of battery chargers.
Let's set up a charging station near the cots.
Medical Supply Co.
I worked long days with the other volunteers to help make sure people's basic needs were met.
Mr. Dominguez and his family will need to go to a shelter for people with medical needs.
Meanwhile, Brian was trying to cope with everyday life...
How is Michelle doing at the convention center?
I don't know.
My cell phone just ran out of power.
Electrical outages continue all over Houston.
Ugh! This has all gone bad, and I'm sick of canned food.
Guess I'll try my luck at the store.
BUZZZZZZZZ

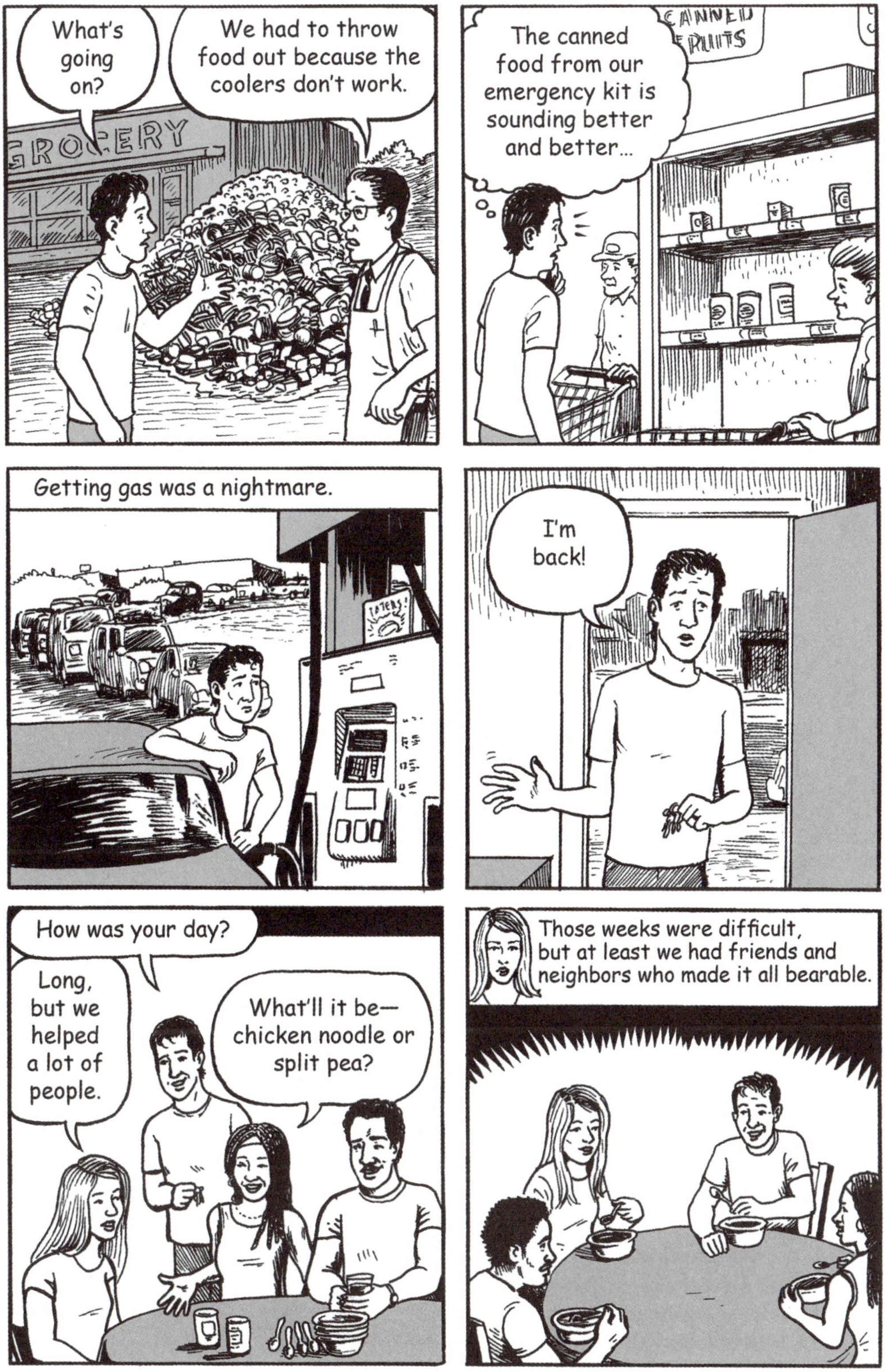
What's going on?
We had to throw food out because the coolers don't work.
GROCERY
The canned food from our emergency kit is sounding better and better...
CANNED FRUITS
Getting gas was a nightmare.
I'm back!
How was your day?
Long, but we helped a lot of people.
What'll it be—chicken noodle or split pea?
Those weeks were difficult, but at least we had friends and neighbors who made it all bearable.

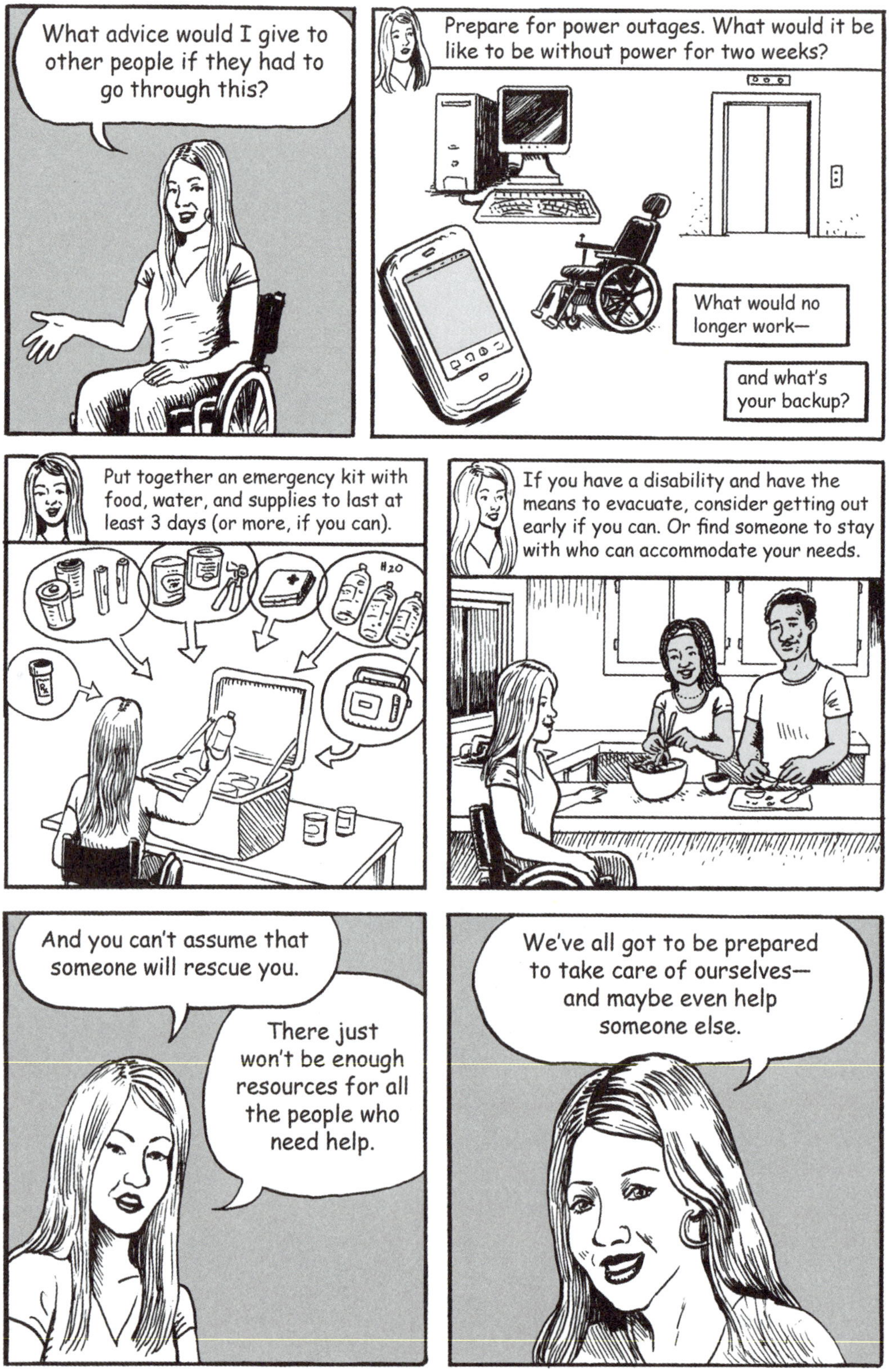
What advice would I give to other people if they had to go through this?
Prepare for power outages. What would it be like to be without power for two weeks?
What would no longer work—
and what's your backup?
Put together an emergency kit with food, water, and supplies to last at least 3 days (or more, if you can).
H2O
If you have a disability and have the means to evacuate, consider getting out early if you can. Or find someone to stay with who can accommodate your needs.
And you can't assume that someone will rescue you.
There just won't be enough resources for all the people who need help.
We've all got to be prepared to take care of ourselves—and maybe even help someone else.

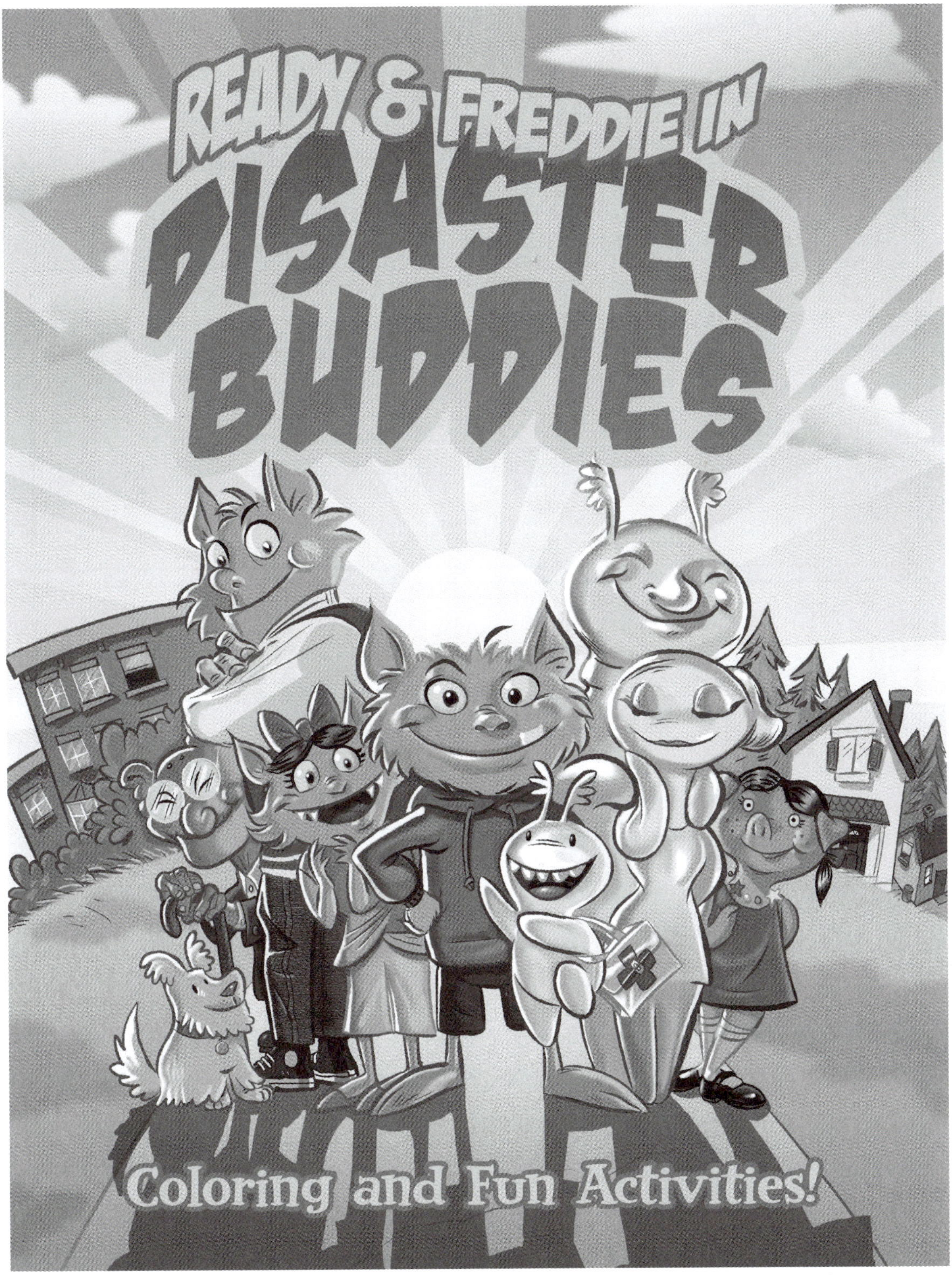
READY & FREDDIE IN
DISASTER BUDDIES
Coloring and Fun Activities!

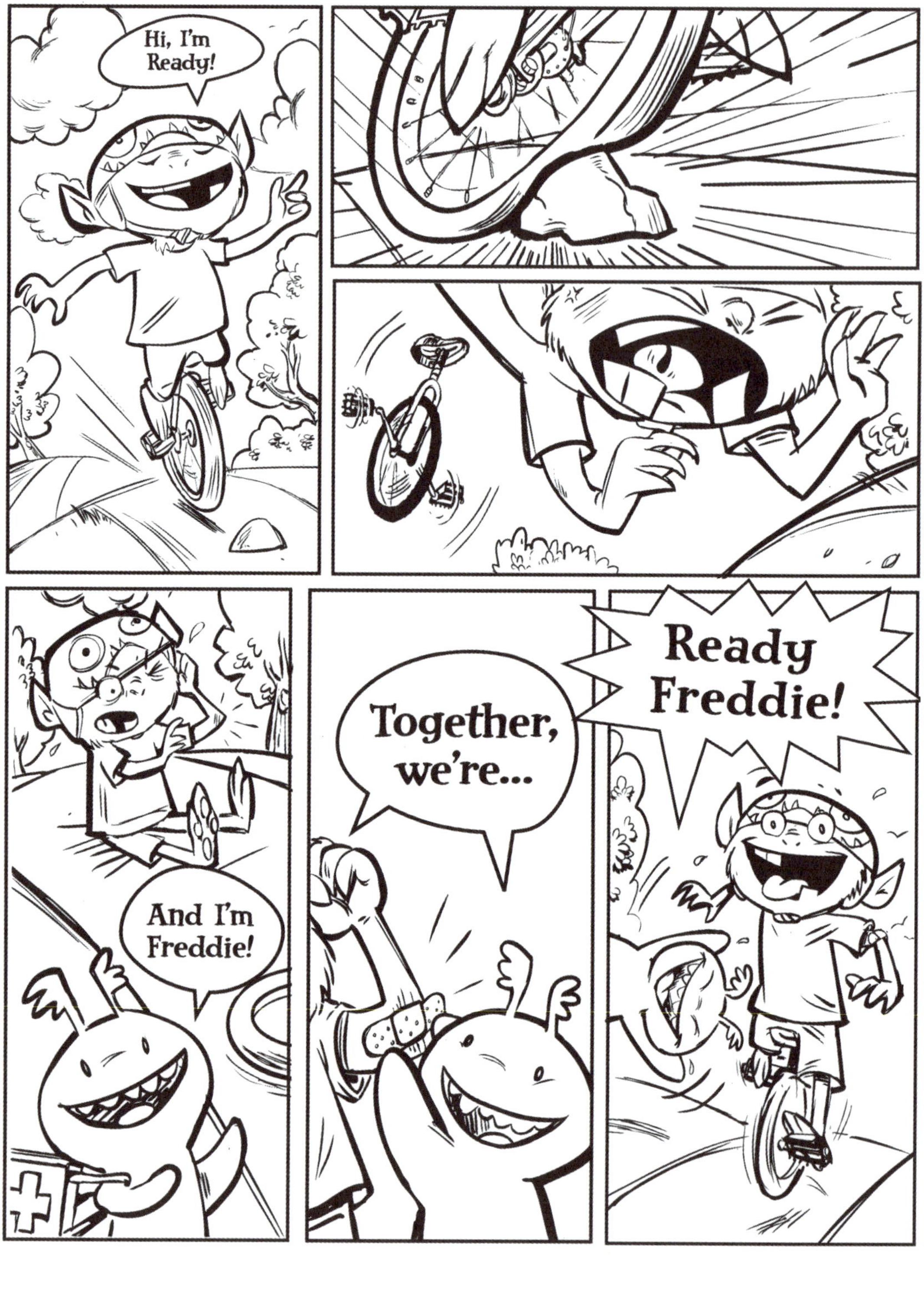
Hi, I'm Ready!
And I'm Freddie!
Together, we're...
Ready Freddie!

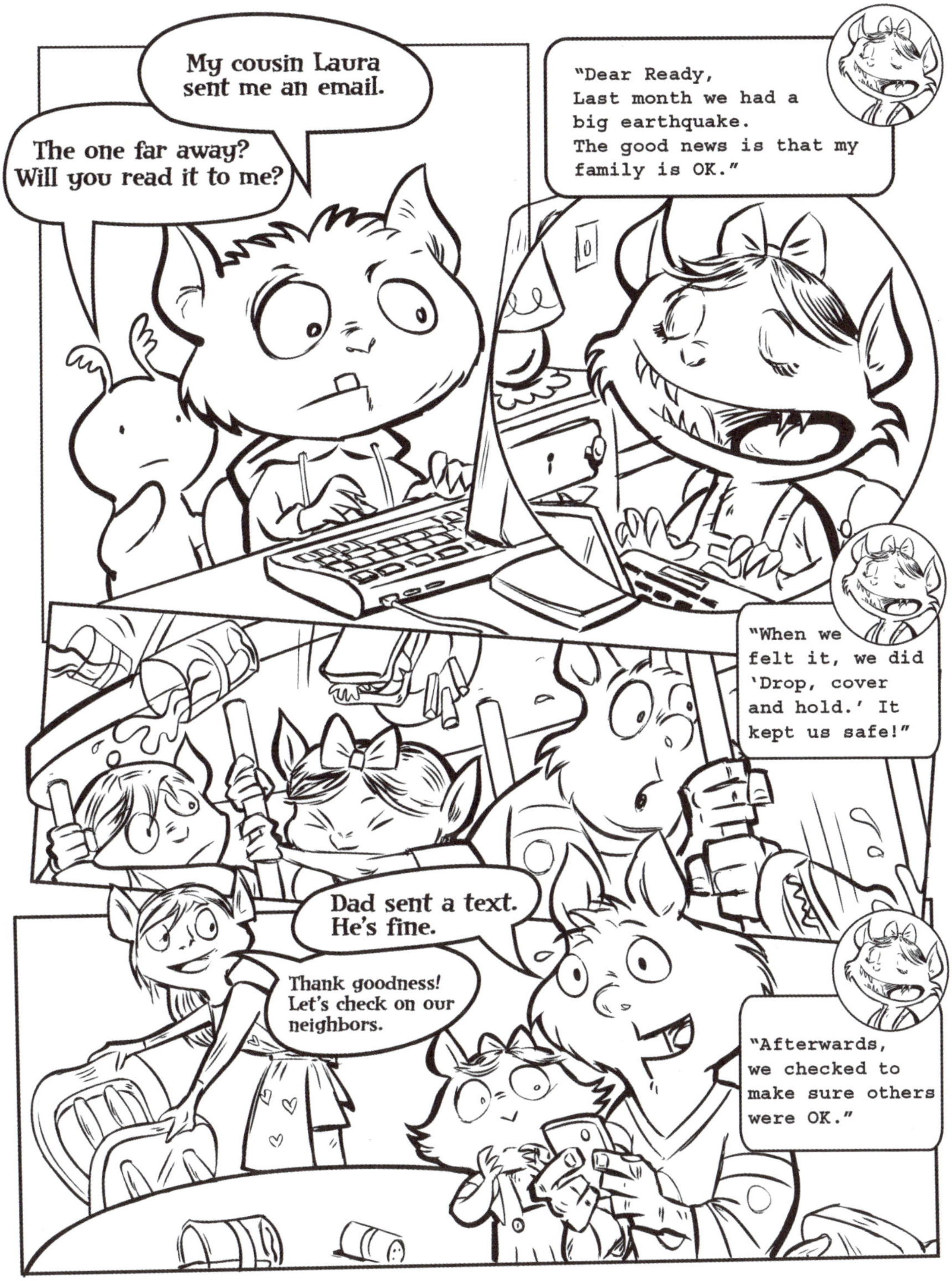

My cousin Laura sent me an email.
The one far away? Will you read it to me?
"Dear Ready,
Last month we had a
big earthquake.
The good news is that my
family is OK."
"When we felt it, we did 'Drop, cover and hold.' It kept us safe!"
Dad sent a text. He's fine.
Thank goodness! Let's check on our neighbors.
"Afterwards, we checked to make sure others were OK."

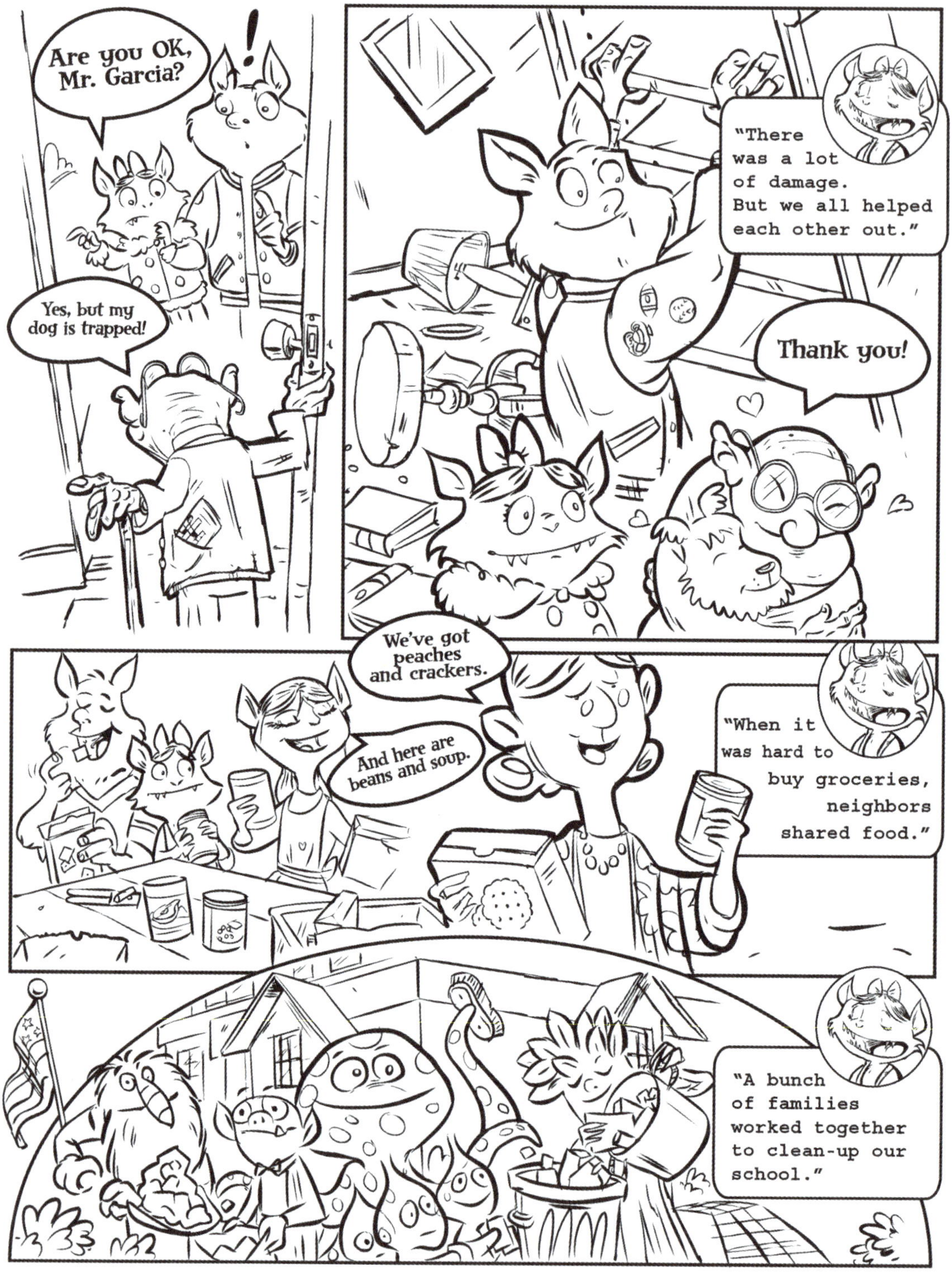
Are you OK, Mr. Garcia?
!
Yes, but my dog is trapped!
"There was a lot of damage. But we all helped each other out."
Thank you!
We've got peaches and crackers.
And here are beans and soup.
"When it was hard to buy groceries, neighbors shared food."
"A bunch of families worked together to clean-up our school."

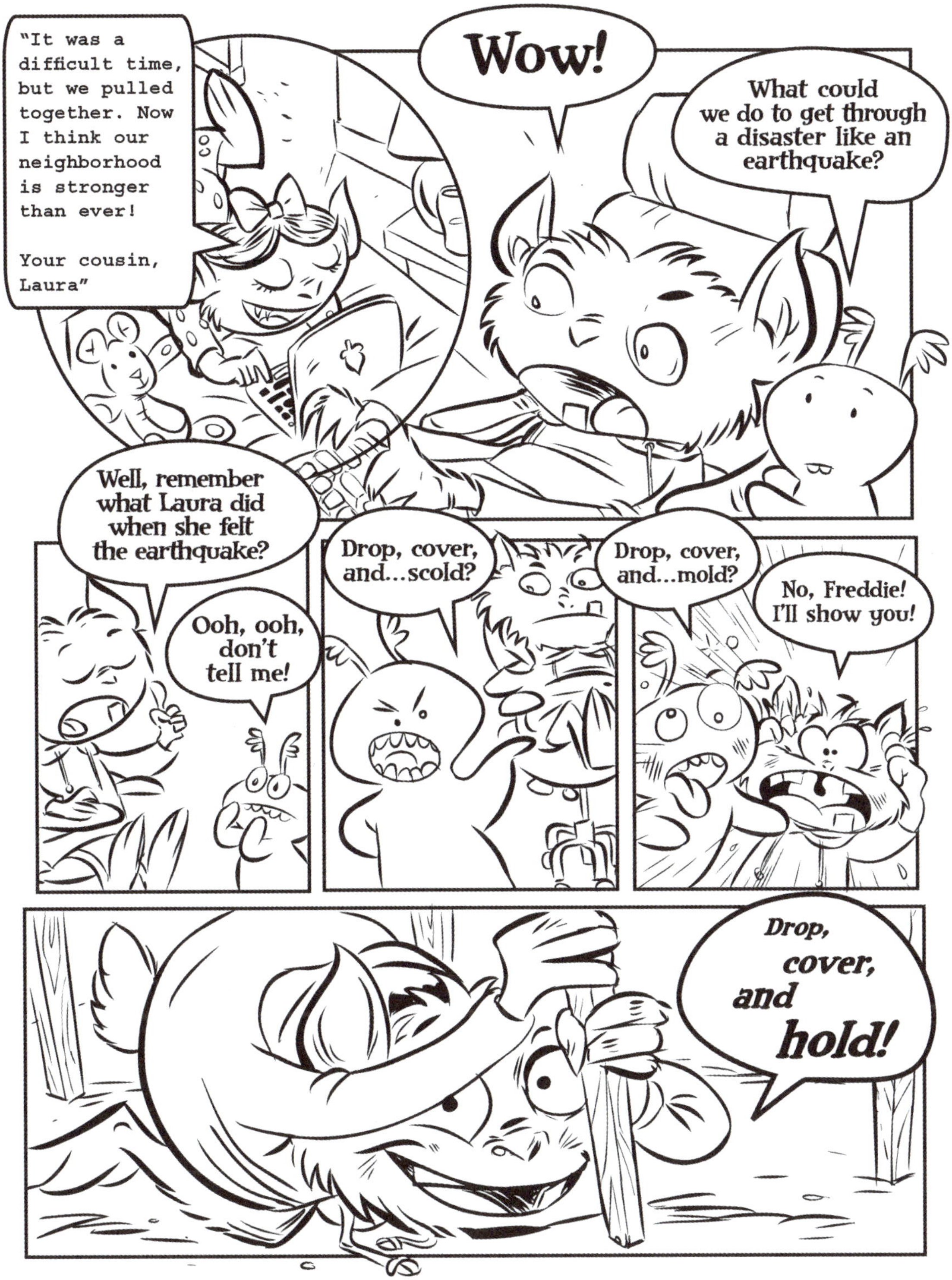
"It was a difficult time, but we pulled together. Now I think our neighborhood is stronger than ever!

Your cousin, Laura"
Wow!
What could we do to get through a disaster like an earthquake?
Well, remember what Laura did when she felt the earthquake?
Ooh, ooh, don't tell me!
Drop, cover, and...scold?
Drop, cover, and...mold?
No, Freddie! I'll show you!
Drop, cover, and hold!

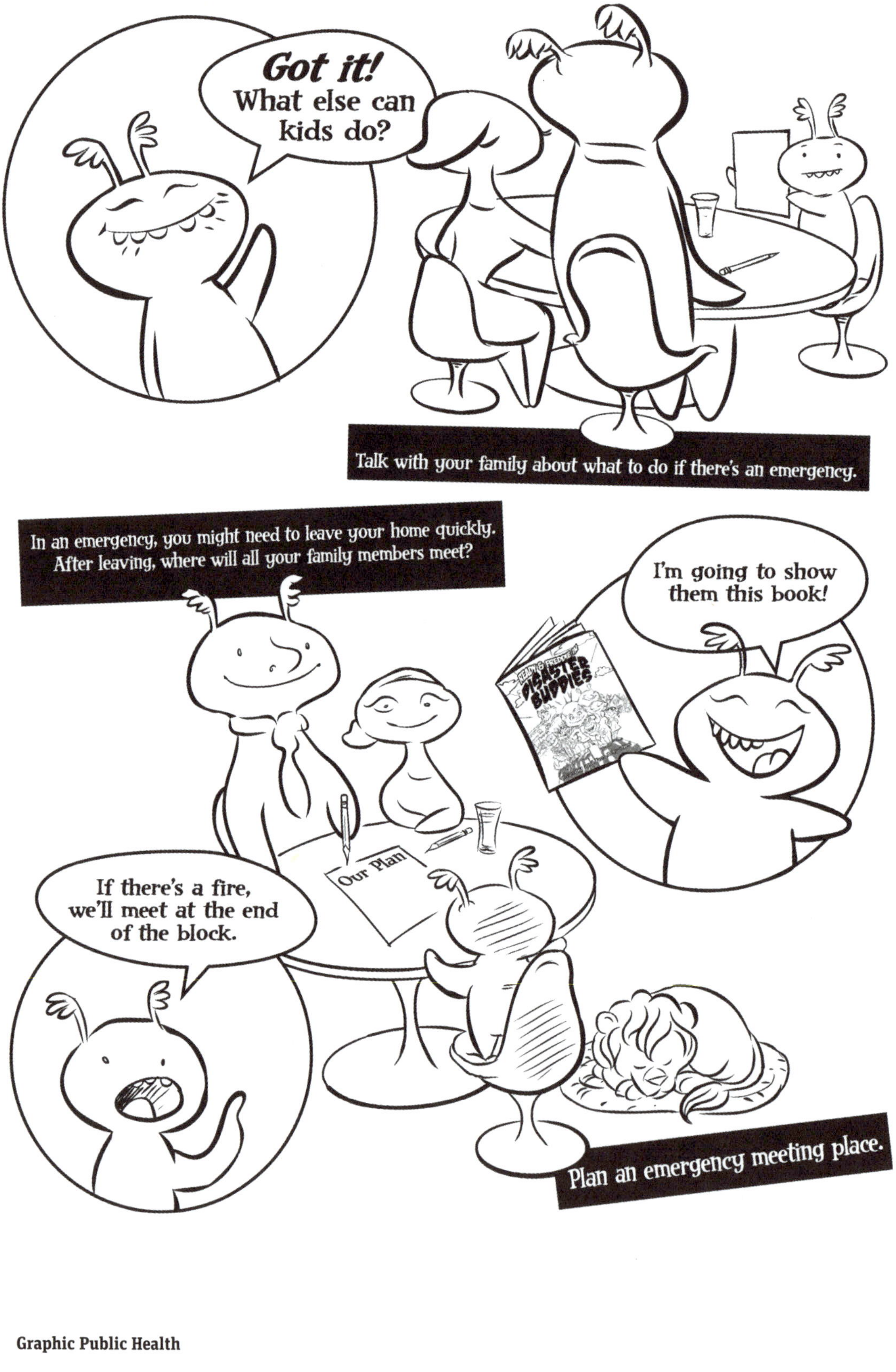
Got it! What else can kids do?
Talk with your family about what to do if there's an emergency.
In an emergency, you might need to leave your home quickly. After leaving, where will all your family members meet?
I'm going to show them this book!
Our Plan
If there's a fire, we'll meet at the end of the block.
Plan an emergency meeting place.

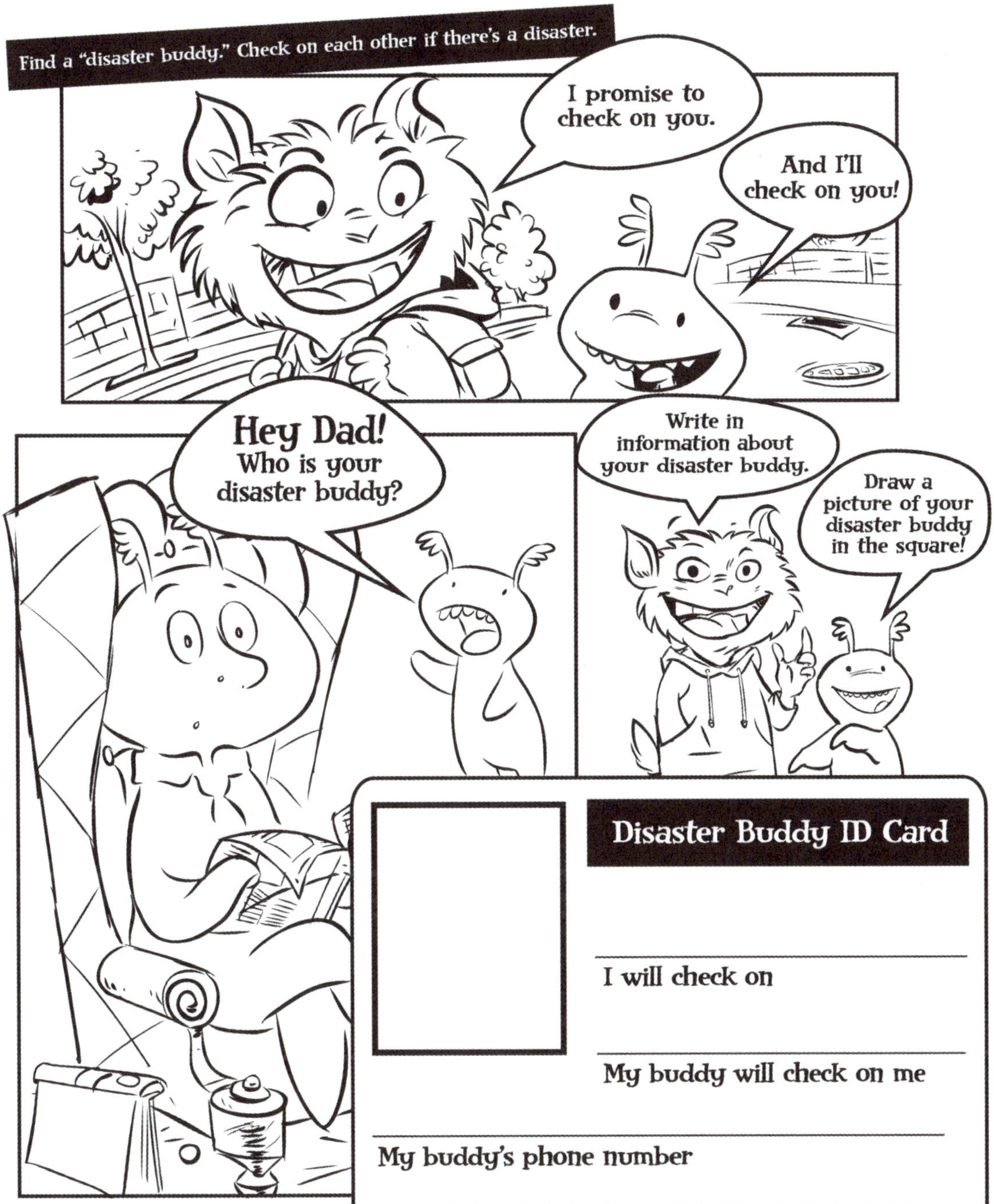
Find a "disaster buddy." Check on each other if there's a disaster.
I promise to check on you.
And I'll check on you!
Hey Dad! Who is your disaster buddy?
Write in information about your disaster buddy.
Draw a picture of your disaster buddy in the square!

Disaster Buddy ID Card

I will check on

My buddy will check on me

My buddy's phone number

My buddy's address

My buddy's email (or family email)

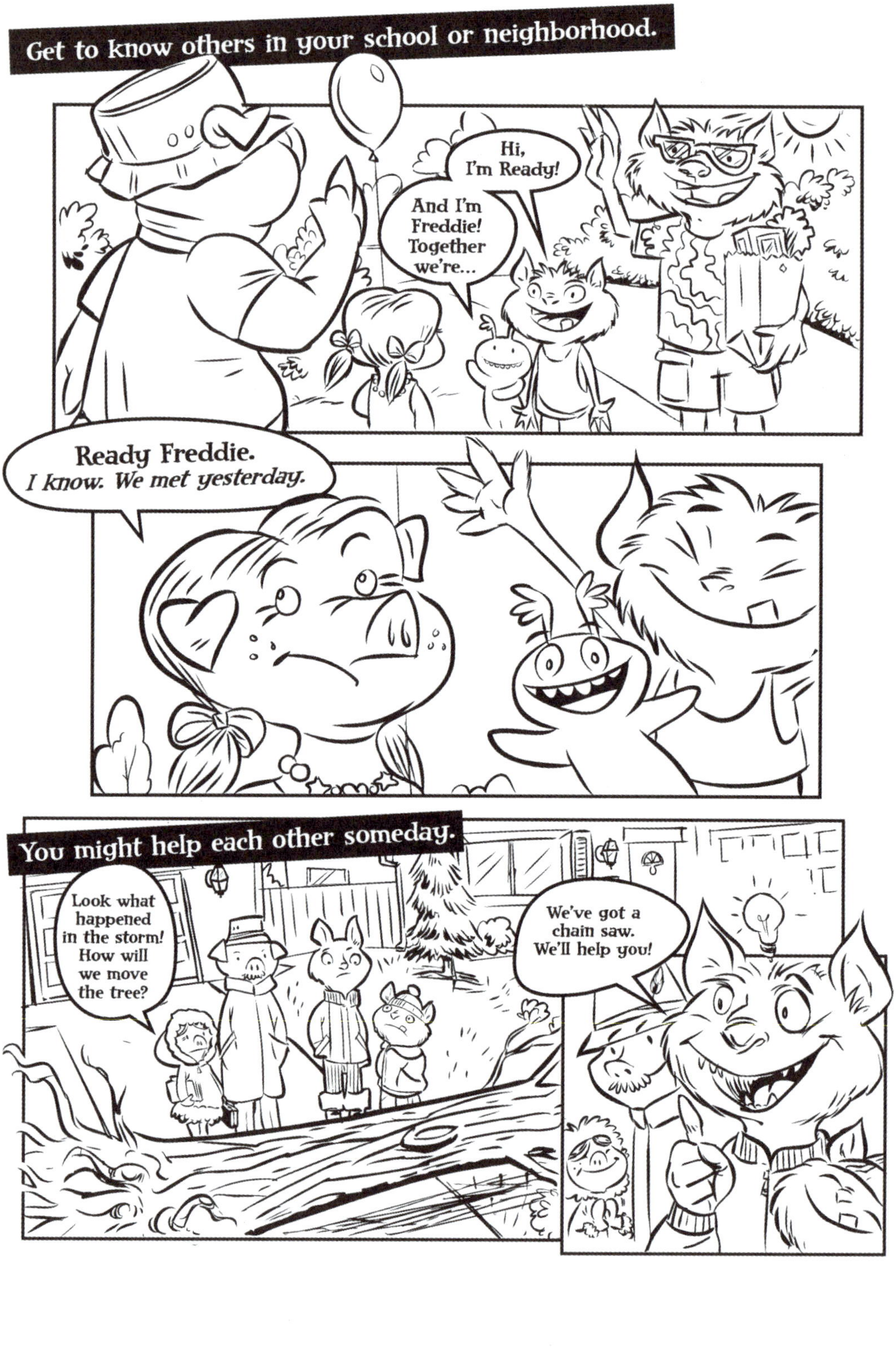

Get to know others in your school or neighborhood.
Hi, I'm Ready!
And I'm Freddie! Together we're...
Ready Freddie.
I know. We met yesterday.
You might help each other someday.
Look what happened in the storm! How will we move the tree?
We've got a chain saw. We'll help you!

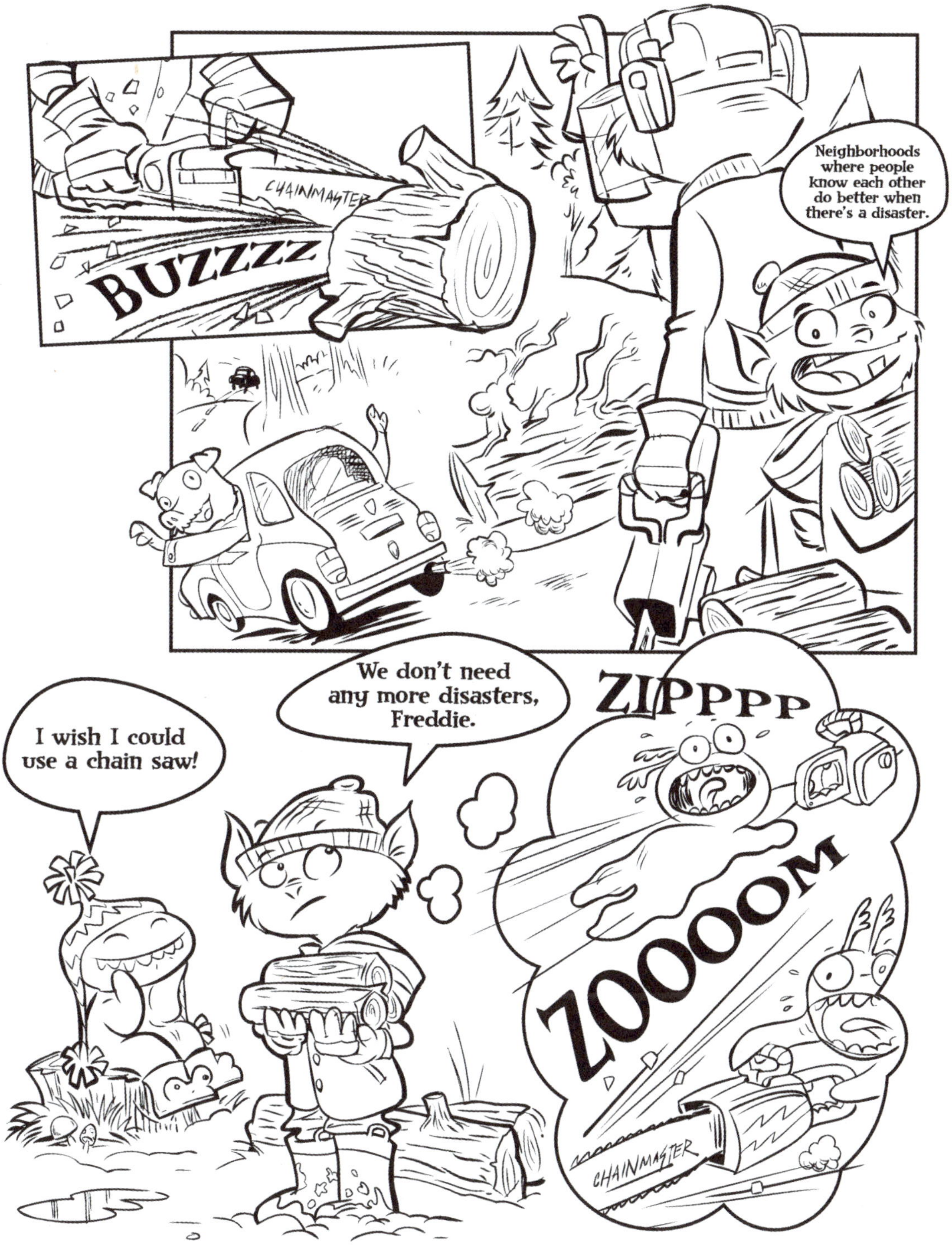
CHAINMASTER
BUZZZZ
Neighborhoods where people know each other do better when there's a disaster.
I wish I could use a chain saw!
We don't need any more disasters, Freddie.
ZIPPPP
ZOOOOOM
CHAINMASTER

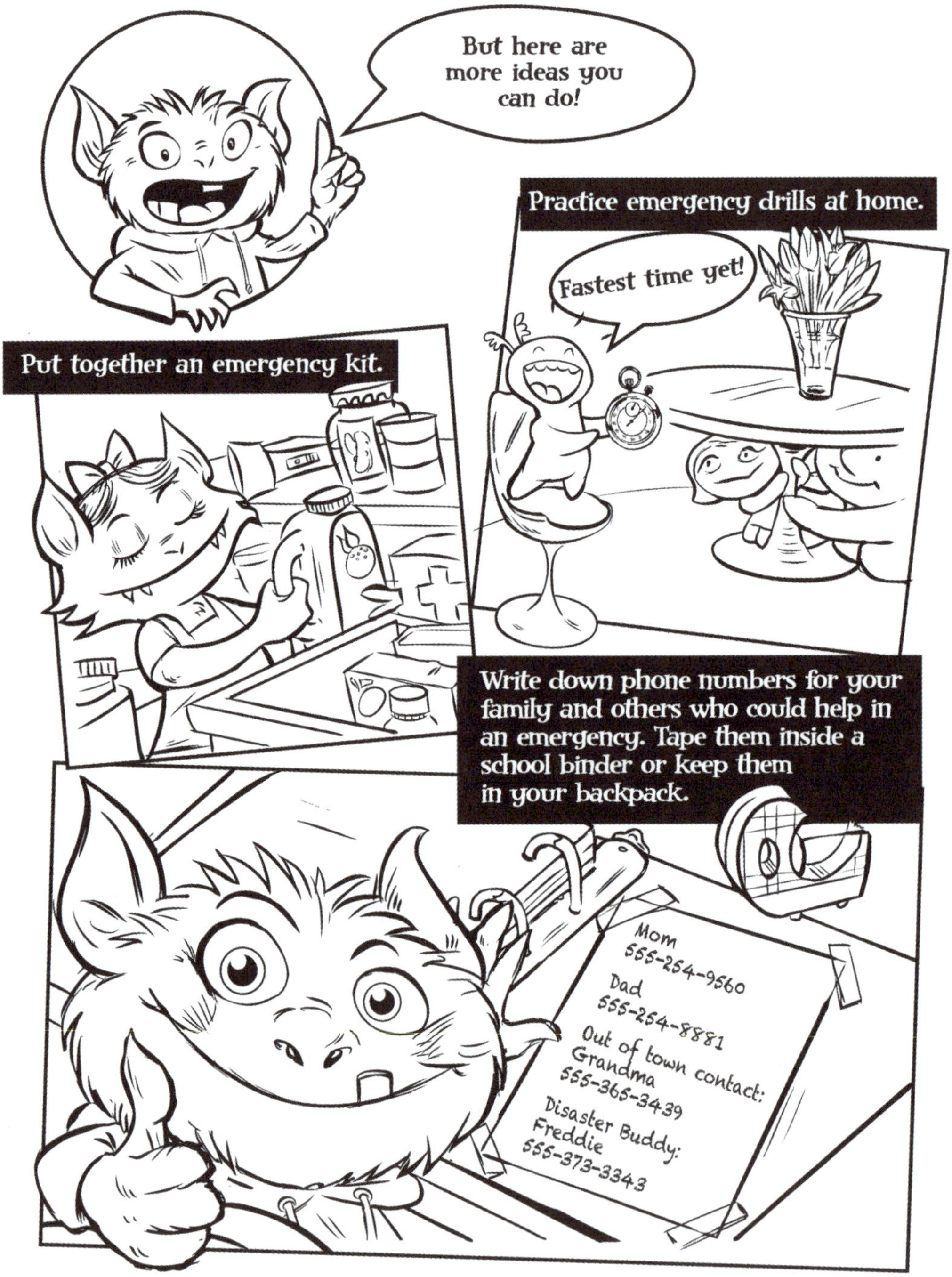

But here are more ideas you can do!
Put together an emergency kit.
Practice emergency drills at home.
Fastest time yet!
Write down phone numbers for your family and others who could help in an emergency. Tape them inside a school binder or keep them in your backpack.
Mom
555-254-9560
Dad
555-254-8881
Out of town contact:
Grandma
555-365-3439
Disaster Buddy:
Freddie
555-373-3343

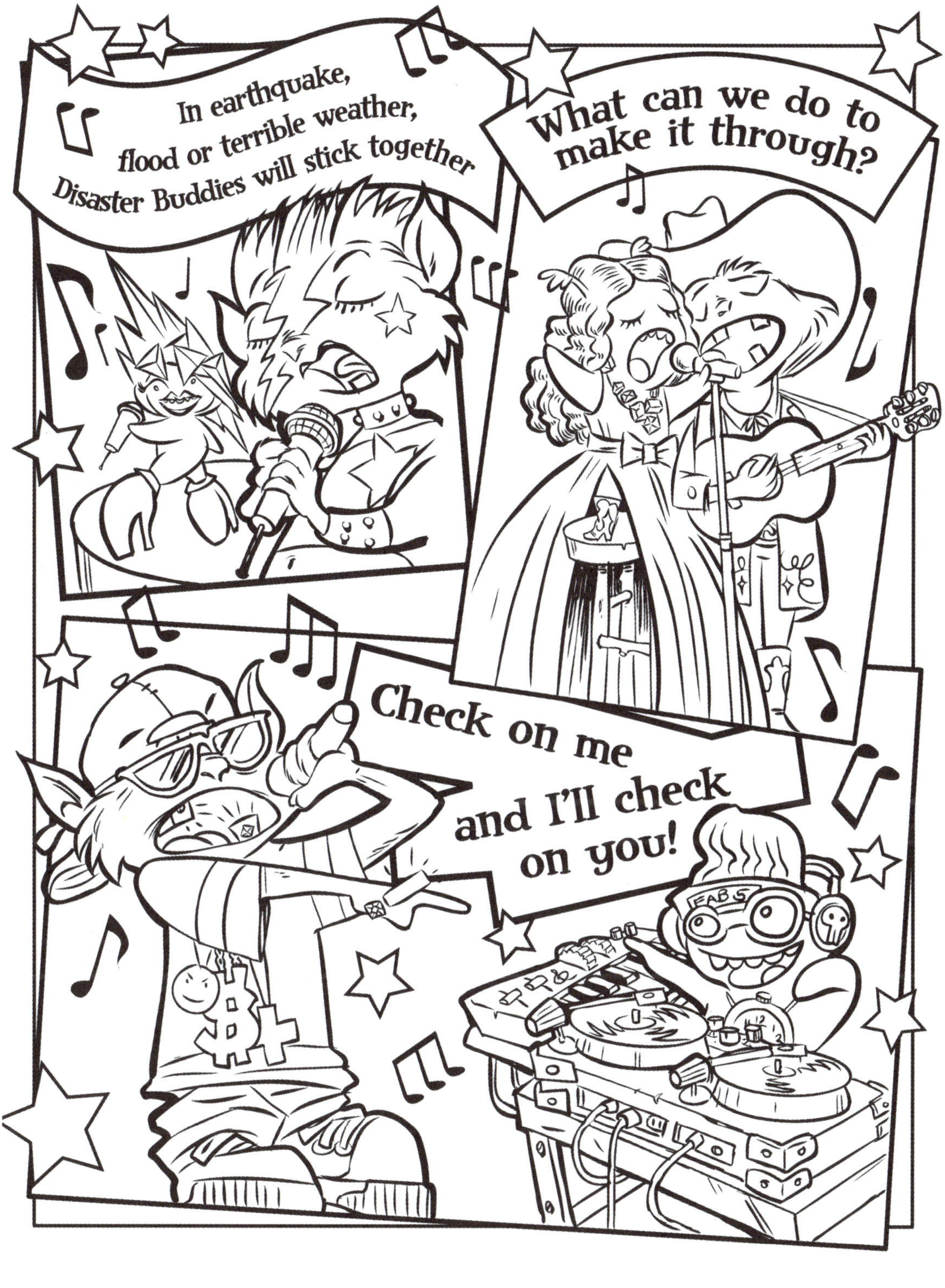
In earthquake, flood or terrible weather, Disaster Buddies will stick together
What can we do to make it through?
Check on me and I'll check on you!
FABS

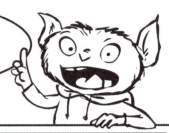

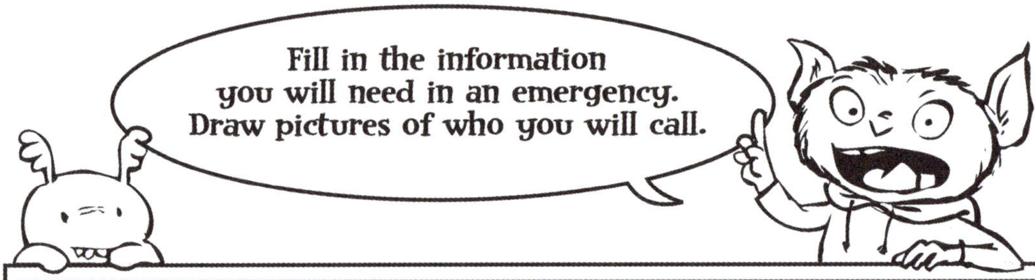

Fill in the information
you will need in an emergency.
Draw pictures of who you will call.

Emergency Contact Information

My phone number:

_____

My address:

_____

_____

ME

Phone numbers of people in my family:

_____ _____ _____

_____ _____ _____

Discussion

Outbreaks. Rabid bats. Lead in water. Health impacts from severe weather, climate change, and earthquakes. These kinds of topics are my specialty within health communications. If it freaks people out, that's when I get to work. In the jargon of public health, we call it risk communication.

Risk communication is the subset of health communications that deals with urgent, emerging health threats. The goal of risk communication is to help people understand the hazards they face and make informed decisions to protect their health during times of high stress. And since this is my area of expertise, I first experimented with comics to communicate about the scary situations.

No Ordinary Flu: Visualizing a Pandemic

In 2007, public health officials were worried that the H5N1 strain of avian flu that was killing large populations of birds in Asia and around the world would jump to humans and become a pandemic flu strain. I was working on public outreach about pandemic flu and trying to promote actions in case of a severe, worldwide pandemic. I found that people had a hard time wrapping their heads around a potentially dire public health emergency that they had never experienced before—at the time, most had never heard of a flu pandemic. In our pre-COVID-19 world, people had a hard time believing that the flu could really be that bad, so there wasn't enough concern to motivate preparations for a catastrophic flu emergency.

However, risk communications specialists like Barbara Reynolds, then at the CDC, found that people engaged with the topic if you told them stories about the terrible influenza pandemic of 1918. The real-life stories were often filled with as much epic drama and heartache as any fictional account, yet those who had lived through it often didn't pass down these stories in their families. When people heard about how the 1918 pandemic played out through personal stories—how everyday life came to a halt, with much of the workforce sick, hospitals overflowing, and schools and public places closed—this formerly nebulous threat felt much more concrete. Reynolds argued that once people accept that severe influenza pandemics can happen, it opens up conversation about the possibility of another pandemic of that scale and what can be done to prepare.

At the time, I had just read Scott McCloud's *Understanding Comics* and was struck by the idea of creating a comic book about the 1918 pandemic as a way of communicating about the current risk. I contacted Seattle artist David Lasky, whose style of drawing was well suited to portraying the turn of the century. (This would be even more apparent in his Eisner Award–winning graphic novel, *The Carter Family: Remember This Song*, which wouldn't be published for another five years.) In our first meeting, to make sure that he could capture the pathos of the pandemic with sensitivity, I asked Lasky whether he was familiar with the 1918 "Spanish Flu" pandemic. Lasky related the story of his great-grandmother, who died from flu in 1918, and his great-grandfather, who left his children in an orphanage after his wife's death. In his deliberate, quiet way of speaking, Lasky explained that his family still felt the reverberations of that traumatic period of their history. Even though I was a novice comics writer, I knew I had found the perfect artist.

Comics Make the Unfamiliar Concrete

By the time I met Lasky, I had already written and storyboarded a draft of the comic to get buy-in within my department, where some were skeptical of the genre's ability to provide serious health information. Lasky refined my visual ideas, creating images that reinforced the suddenness and severity of the 1918 flu pandemic. Scenes of deserted streets, dialogue about dire situations like the shortage of coffins, and the grief on the faces of the characters vividly demonstrated the enormous disruption caused by the pandemic with a limited amount of exposition. The images illustrated the scale and scope of a severe pandemic—and reinforced how it could happen again.

Comics Support Mental Rehearsal

The images in *No Ordinary Flu* were designed to facilitate "mental rehearsal," a process of thinking through expected outcomes in advance. Mental rehearsal can help make decision-making easier in times of stress and can prepare the public for unusual measures that may be necessary in crisis situations. At the time that we developed *No Ordinary Flu*, we had no idea that these images would also preview what would unfold in a global coronavirus pandemic over a decade later.

No Ordinary Flu depicted possible scenarios for a modern-day pandemic—including social distancing measures, such as a closed school and a cancelled sporting event—to increase awareness of possible health orders for audiences who were still years from experiencing COVID-19. An illustration of an overcrowded emergency room accompanies text about how medical care may be difficult to access, followed by a conversation between health care providers about how illness has reduced their workforce. These panels were all designed to help readers grasp what to expect in a catastrophic pandemic. The final panels model what people can do to cope with a severe pandemic; here, the illustrations of stocked goods and neighbors dropping off supplies demonstrate possible actions more efficiently than lists for emergency kits or detailed explanations can.

A Comic for Mental Rehearsal of the Unthinkable

What to Expect at a Medication Center is another comic to encourage mental rehearsal of an unfamiliar emergency situation. This comic was created for use in an incident like a bioterrorist attack or rapidly spreading outbreak that requires federal deployment of medical countermeasures (jargon for emergency medications or vaccinations). Ever since anthrax was sent through the US mail as a form of terrorism in 2001, public health departments have made plans to issue such medications quickly—in the case of anthrax, entire populations might need to receive life-saving antibiotics within forty-eight hours of exposure.

It would take an extraordinary emergency for medical countermeasures to be issued. These kinds of events are low on the probability of happening but high on the level of upset they could generate. In such an unfamiliar and dire situation, people may balk at taking medication supplied by the government. Some may question the need to get the medication because they harbor mistrust of the government or of pharmaceuticals, and others may feel intense anxiety about getting their own supply.

Outreach on such emergencies is not likely to be effective if delivered *before* such an emergency happens. People are unlikely to retain the details of what to do if that scenario is not yet a reality. *What to Expect at a Medication Center* was created for the "just-in-time" moment, immediately following notification that an emergency situation has emerged. In the window of time before the health department has received deliveries of emergency medication, this comic could be widely distributed across social media and news platforms to show people what types of locations will have the medications, such as pharmacies, workplaces, and community centers.

In illustrating how community centers may be used as places to pick up medications, David Lasky referenced photographs from actual emergency drills so that it would look as close to the real thing as possible. The illustration of the long lines that people may encounter help sets expectations, but it also conveys a sense of orderliness and calm within the medication center. Further thought went into the characterizations of the staff shown at medication centers, striking a balance between the seriousness of the situation and the staff's friendliness and attentiveness to the people at the center. Overall, the comic aims to capture a feeling of competence so that people will feel confident that there is a strong system in place to respond to the emergency (fig. 2.1).

An unfamiliar crisis event with potential for serious or even fatal health outcomes will induce high levels of stress. When people are under stress, their brains are flooded with stress hormones that make it hard for them to process information and make decisions. The accessibility of information in comics may make it easier for people to absorb critical information and take action quickly. With this in mind, one panel in *What to Expect at a Medication Center* simply models a person getting ready to

STATE CHAMPIONS
Step 3: Get Vaccine
Step 2: Show Form

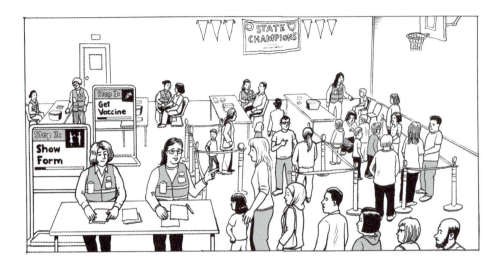

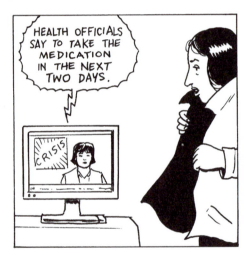

Fig. 2.1. This panel from *What to Expect at a Medication Center* was designed to help people with mental rehearsal for a sudden public health emergency that requires people to get medications or vaccinations quickly. Artwork by David Lasky. Courtesy of Public Health—Seattle & King County.

HEALTH OFFICIALS SAY TO TAKE THE MEDICATION IN THE NEXT TWO DAYS.
CRISIS

Fig. 2.2. When a timely response to a public health message is critical, comics showing what to do may help facilitate quick action. Artwork by David Lasky for *What to Expect at a Medication Center*. Courtesy of Public Health—Seattle & King County.

leave to pick up medication just as the news reports where to go, showing that taking medication in time is of the utmost importance (fig. 2.2).

What to Expect at a Medication Center is at the ready in case it's needed, when there would be insufficient time to develop illustrated communications from scratch. Given the dire type of crisis for which it was created, I hope that it can just stay in the public health toolbox, even if it means that few people ever see the work we put into it.

Comics to Communicate in Stressful Circumstances

Even in circumstances less dire than a medical countermeasure emergency, stress and anxiety can impair people's ability to process information. To overcome the "mental

Stay away from others until the health department says it is safe to go out.
Do NOT do any of the things shown:
Do not ride the bus or use other public transportation.
Do not ride an airplane.
Do not go to work.
Do not go to school.
Do not go to social gatherings.
Do not have visitors in your home.
Do not go to restaurants.
Do not go to the store.

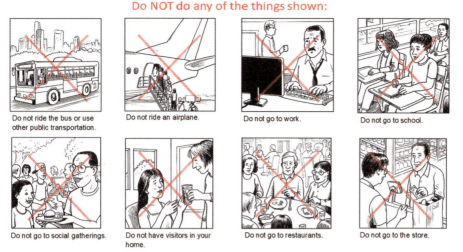

Fig. 2.3. This excerpt from a flyer shows what people should not do when in isolation or quarantine. The flyer was developed to help eliminate confusion for those under quarantine or isolation orders. Artwork by David Lasky for "Staying at Home Fact Sheet." Courtesy of Public Health—Seattle & King County.

noise" that is common when stress hormones kick in, information must be made as easy to comprehend as possible.

Banking on Comics Panels

Isolation and quarantine orders mandate that people stay away from others, with precisely defined parameters for what a person can and cannot do. However, if people can't fully comprehend the guidance for isolation and quarantine, they won't be able to follow the necessary steps to prevent the spread of disease. To make these detailed instructions more easily accessible under stressful circumstances, I worked with David Lasky to create guidance illustrated with comics.

Even without reading the written instructions of what not to do while in isolation or quarantine, the "X" drawn over these panels immediately communicates the message (fig. 2.3). What behaviors are permissible during isolation and quarantine can vary, depending on the nature of the infectious disease and the likelihood of infection, so Lasky created a bank of images that the health department could use in a variety of circumstances. This approach was so well received by the Washington State Department of Health that it later commissioned Lasky to create a bank of over three hundred images depicting symptoms of illness and health behaviors, which health departments in the state could use as needed in their health communications.

COVID-19 VACCINE
COMMUNICATION CARD
Health
YES
NO
? I don't know
A B C D E F G H I J K L M N O
P Q R S T U V W X Y Z
0 1 2 3 4 5 6 7 8 9
HOURS
DAYS
Tell the provider all of your medical conditions, including:
received a COVID-19 vaccine
allergies
fever
bleeding disorder
on blood thinner
pregnant or planning pregnancy
breastfeeding
immunocompromised or on medicine affecting immune system
Don't get vaccine if you:
are younger than 16 years of age
had a severe allergic reaction after a previous dose of this vaccine
had a severe allergic reaction to any ingredient of this vaccine
Possible side effects:
injection site pain
injection site swelling
injection site redness
muscle or joint pain
swollen lymph nodes
fever
chills
tiredness
nausea
feeling unwell

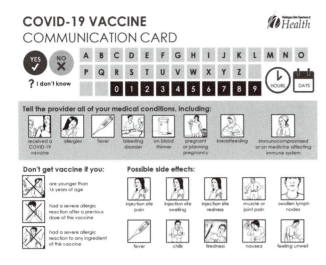

Fig. 2.4. The Washington State Department of Health used images from a comics image bank to put together a tool to help vaccination site staff communicate with people with lower literacy or those whose English is limited. Artwork by David Lasky.

Comics During COVID-19

The premade bank of comics from Lasky was put to good use when the first reported case of COVID-19 in the United States arrived through Sea-Tac International Airport in King County, Washington. Public health communicators across the state used illustrations from the comics bank in the first messages for Americans who might have been exposed. The comics also surfaced in Washington State Department of Health materials that were used at COVID-19 vaccination sites to assist with communicating with patients from many language communities (fig. 2.4).

Stay Safe at Home: Comics to Support Older Adults

During the COVID-19 pandemic, one of the communications gaps identified was information specifically for older adults who were more at risk from coronavirus. People over age sixty needed to understand the urgency of staying away from others, and they also needed tips for coping with their increasing isolation. At the same time, many essential workers who had exposure to others in places like hospitals, warehouses, and grocery stores also lived in multigenerational homes; they wanted crucial information about how to protect any older adults who lived with them. Leaders in immigrant communities requested easy-to-understand guidance that was not entirely dependent on the written word so that those with lower literacy in their spoken language could grasp what they needed to do. These community leaders also provided details about daily activities that might put elders in multigenerational homes at risk as well as input on what safety measures were feasible and relevant for the families in their communities.

Kelly Froh, a cartoonist and the Executive Director of Short Run Comix and Arts in Seattle, was the ideal person to help develop materials to reach older audiences. From teaching art workshops for seniors and from her other job, providing in-home services to senior clients, Froh has expertise in the needs of seniors and a love of working with older adults. Based on her conversations and interactions with this age group, Froh illustrated ways for older adults to stay active at home, physically and socially. Her trademark loose, witty style imbued the characters with personality, appealing to seniors by depicting them as vibrant and independent rather than as merely vulnerable.

The resulting *Stay Safe at Home* comics created a flexible communications tool. They appeared in newsletters published in several languages and inserted into food boxes delivered to homebound elderly or mailed directly to their homes. The comic also adapted well to platforms like Instagram and Facebook to reach the growing numbers of people over sixty using social media. When advocates in immigrant communities requested more accessible content via video, Froh adapted the comics into short, stop-action animations with voiceovers in languages that are primarily spoken but not read, like Somali and Tongan.

"A Very COVID Holiday"

As the end of 2020 drew near, ten months since the first case of COVID-19 in the United States, people were weary from trying to keep up with public health measures like wearing masks and social distancing. Cases were beginning to rise steeply in November, and the holiday season was approaching. As health experts promoted cautionary warnings about the dangers of holiday gatherings, the public also needed to hear empathy about their hardships. People often make decisions based on how they *feel* rather than what they know. If public health warnings were to have any credibility, people needed to know that the public health department understood the considerable sacrifice being asked of them. To take a more empathetic approach to public health messaging, I wrote and drew "A Very COVID Holiday" about my own personal dilemmas related to holiday gatherings.

The narrative focuses on the emotional pull of being with family members (and concerns for their social isolation) and the importance of protecting them from a potentially devasting virus. The comic encourages other ways of being together, such as connecting online or going for a walk outside rather than a meal indoors. When the comic appeared on the blog and Instagram of the King County health department, the high level of engagement with our followers suggested that it resonated, prompting a direct mailing of the comic on a postcard sent to residents in advance of the December holidays.

Comics to Motivate Emergency Preparedness

One of the common tasks of risk communication specialists is to promote emergency preparedness, and it is one of the most thankless parts of the job. Few people get excited about emergency preparedness, and those who do are usually already well prepared for disasters. Alarming people with descriptions of the destruction that disasters could wreak often backfires—people can feel overwhelmed at the thought, or prefer to tune out scary warnings, or feel that there's nothing they can do to prevent an act of nature. I've looked to comics for alternative ways to engage people on emergency preparedness.

Survivor Tales: Comics to Tell Authentic Stories of Resilience

In 2009, a new series of comics was inspired by the public fascination surrounding a news story about an airline pilot who safely landed a disabled commercial airplane on the Hudson River in the dead of winter. A near disaster was averted, and 155 people survived. The public just could not get enough of Captain Chesley "Sully" Sullenberger, the hero who used his wits and skill to save lives. With Captain Sully's example in mind for emergency preparedness promotion, I decided to focus on survival and resilience rather than the potential bad outcomes of disasters, and graphic memoir offered a way to share what became the *Survivor Tales* project.

Graphic memoir is my favorite genre of comics. A person's intimate experience, expressed from their perspective, offers a depth of insight into what they've been through and encourages empathy for their situation. For the *Survivor Tales* project, memoirs from actual survivors of major disasters served as the basis for a series of comic books: one on earthquakes, one on floods, and one on hurricanes. For each story, I interviewed a survivor, paying particular attention to the parts of their stories that highlighted how friends, family, and neighbors helped one another.

The resulting comic books offer authentic accounts of how people handled crisis, as told through the survivors' words and memories. David Lasky, my collaborator once again, did careful research, even traveling to the site of a flooded farm belonging to one of the survivors to make sure he captured the feel of the place. The stories emphasize community resilience by showing the myriad of ways in which people helped one another. Each story ends with the survivor offering advice, giving the emergency preparedness tips an authenticity that someone who has lived through the experience can lend.

Ready Freddie! and *Disaster Buddies*

Children are one of the rare audiences that actually like emergency preparedness. Working with a group of emergency managers in King County, Washington, I wrote two comic books for elementary school–aged kids, *Ready Freddie!* and *Disaster Buddies*, to give them ideas to help their families be ready for disasters and to encourage them to involve their parents in their efforts.

These books aim to avoid the overly wholesome, goody-two-shoes look and feel of educational materials that can be the kiss of death with kids. They credit kids' own capabilities to do the important work of preparing for emergencies. These books also emphasize actions that children could feasibly do to protect their families, rather than relying on superheroes or superpowers. The main characters, "Ready" and "Freddie," are two slightly wacky monster children who, even without supernatural abilities, can still play an instrumental role in getting their households ready for disasters. Drawn by artist Thomas Webb and his team at Bauer Graphics in Portland, these two monsters are infused with delightful irreverence and a lovable goofiness. At the same time, they serve as confident leaders in their families.

The first comic book, *Ready Freddie!*, models for kids and their families how they can protect themselves in earthquakes and how to prepare for electrical outages and storms. The drawing activities included in the book help children think about what they could put in their emergency kits and where they would meet their families if they ever became separated.

Disaster Buddies, the sequel to *Ready Freddie!*, focuses on preparedness information that can be used by people who don't have the ability to purchase large amounts of emergency supplies. Focus groups with Spanish-speaking parents indicated that they wanted to be prepared for emergencies but lacked the resources to invest in emergency supply kits when they were concerned about just having enough food on the table under normal circumstances. What they felt was more practical was the idea of creating emergency contacts and communications plans for reaching loved ones. Additionally, they felt that encouraging neighbors to help one another was culturally appropriate, but they explained that the language barrier between themselves and other members of their community made it difficult to meet their neighbors.

Disaster Buddies, then, was created to model how children can play a role in connecting neighboring families to one another. The comic book encourages children to identify their disaster buddy (creating a disaster buddy ID card) and shows the characters asking their parents who their disaster buddies are and introducing themselves to the kid next door. The visuals in *Disaster Buddies* demonstrate that connection can begin with a friendly wave to the neighbors and later lead to neighborly assistance between households. In the parlance of risk communication, the *Disaster Buddies* comic book is a tool to foster community resilience, with children as the catalyst.

Risk Communication Comics: A Natural Fit

In 2008, when I first proposed a comic book to communicate the risks of a severe influenza pandemic, I had to convince my public health colleagues that the medium would work for this serious topic. At the time, it may have seemed an oddball approach for those unfamiliar with the breadth and depth of the genre.

But our forays into comics found that they are highly adaptable to both the information demands and empathetic approaches needed for effective risk communication. The combination of image, words, and sequence makes the comics medium uniquely suitable for communicating in times of crisis, when critical life and safety messages must be easy to comprehend.[1] They can highlight aspects of emergency situations that resonate, and they can engage people through stories about survival, interpersonal bonding, heroism, and hardship. In the years since we published *No Ordinary Flu*, we've lived through a pandemic that closely resembles that first comic book, and we've found that comics are a natural fit for risk communication.

3.

Comics for Health Promotion

The Comics

Excerpts from the Don't Hang on to Meds Campaign (2018), King County

87 "Youth Story," from *Don't Hang on to Meds*, written by Meredith Li-Vollmer, artwork by Tatiana Gill, 2018. Courtesy of Public Health—Seattle & King County.

88 "Grandparent Story," from *Don't Hang on to Meds*, written by Meredith Li-Vollmer, artwork by Tatiana Gill, 2018. Courtesy of Public Health—Seattle & King County.

89 "Poison Center Story," from *Don't Hang on to Meds*, written by Meredith Li-Vollmer, artwork by Tatiana Gill, 2018. Courtesy of Public Health—Seattle & King County.

90 "Environment Story," from *Don't Hang on to Meds*, written by Meredith Li-Vollmer, artwork by Tatiana Gill, 2018. Courtesy of Public Health—Seattle & King County.

Lead Poisoning Testing for Children Campaign (2018), Public Health—Seattle & King County

91 *Why Testing for Lead Helps Kids and Their Growing Brains*, written by Meredith Li-Vollmer, artwork by Amy Camber, 2018. Courtesy of Public Health—Seattle & King County.

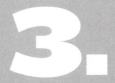

I STARTED TAKING PILLS FROM MY MOM'S MEDICINE CABINET WHEN I WAS 13. I WAS DEALING WITH A LOT OF ANXIETY. PILLS WERE EASY TO GET AND NO ONE SEEMED TO NOTICE.
LATER I TOOK PILLS FROM OTHER PEOPLE'S MEDICINE CABINETS. I STOLE MORE AND MORE OF THE PILLS.
MY PILL USE ENDED UP CREATING A LOT OF PAIN FOR ME AND MY FAMILY. I THINK MY LIFE WOULD'VE BEEN DIFFERENT IF I HADN'T BEEN ABLE TO GET THOSE PILLS SO EASILY.
SOME TEENS THINK MEDICINES ARE SAFE TO EXPERIMENT WITH. SO ANY KID MIGHT TRY THEM. NO ONE SUSPECTED ME.
DEBATE TEAM 1st Place
State Champs Junior Soccer
AND IT MIGHT BE A FRIEND, OR A FAMILY MEMBER WHO TAKES YOUR PILLS WITHOUT YOUR KNOWLEDGE. MY ADVICE? KEEP MEDICINE LOCKED UP.
IF YOU HAVE ANY MEDS YOU AREN'T TAKING OR THEY ARE EXPIRED, GET RID OF THEM AT A LOCAL TAKE-BACK BOX. YOU'RE KEEPING THE PEOPLE AROUND YOU SAFE.
Pharmacy
SAFELY DISPOSE OF MEDICINES
SAFELY DISPOSE OF MEDICINES

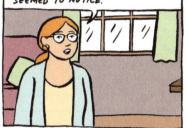

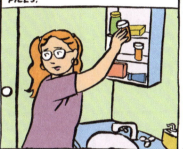

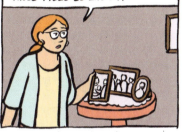

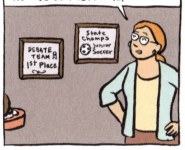

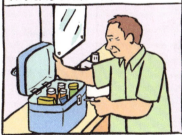

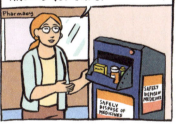

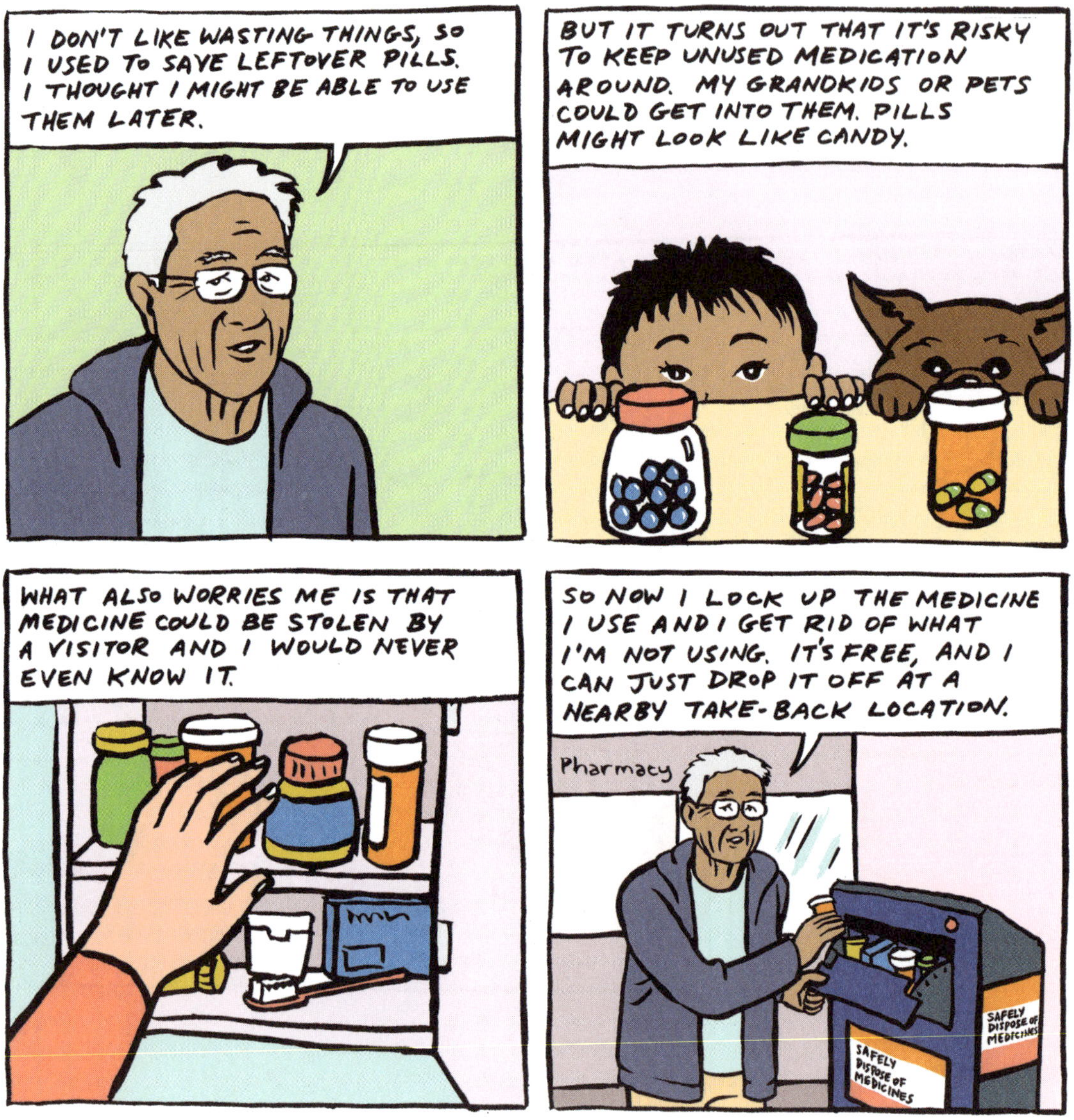
I DON'T LIKE WASTING THINGS, SO I USED TO SAVE LEFTOVER PILLS. I THOUGHT I MIGHT BE ABLE TO USE THEM LATER.
BUT IT TURNS OUT THAT IT'S RISKY TO KEEP UNUSED MEDICATION AROUND. MY GRANDKIDS OR PETS COULD GET INTO THEM. PILLS MIGHT LOOK LIKE CANDY.
WHAT ALSO WORRIES ME IS THAT MEDICINE COULD BE STOLEN BY A VISITOR AND I WOULD NEVER EVEN KNOW IT.
SO NOW I LOCK UP THE MEDICINE I USE AND I GET RID OF WHAT I'M NOT USING. IT'S FREE, AND I CAN JUST DROP IT OFF AT A NEARBY TAKE-BACK LOCATION.
Pharmacy
SAFELY DISPOSE OF MEDICINES
SAFELY DISPOSE OF MEDICINES

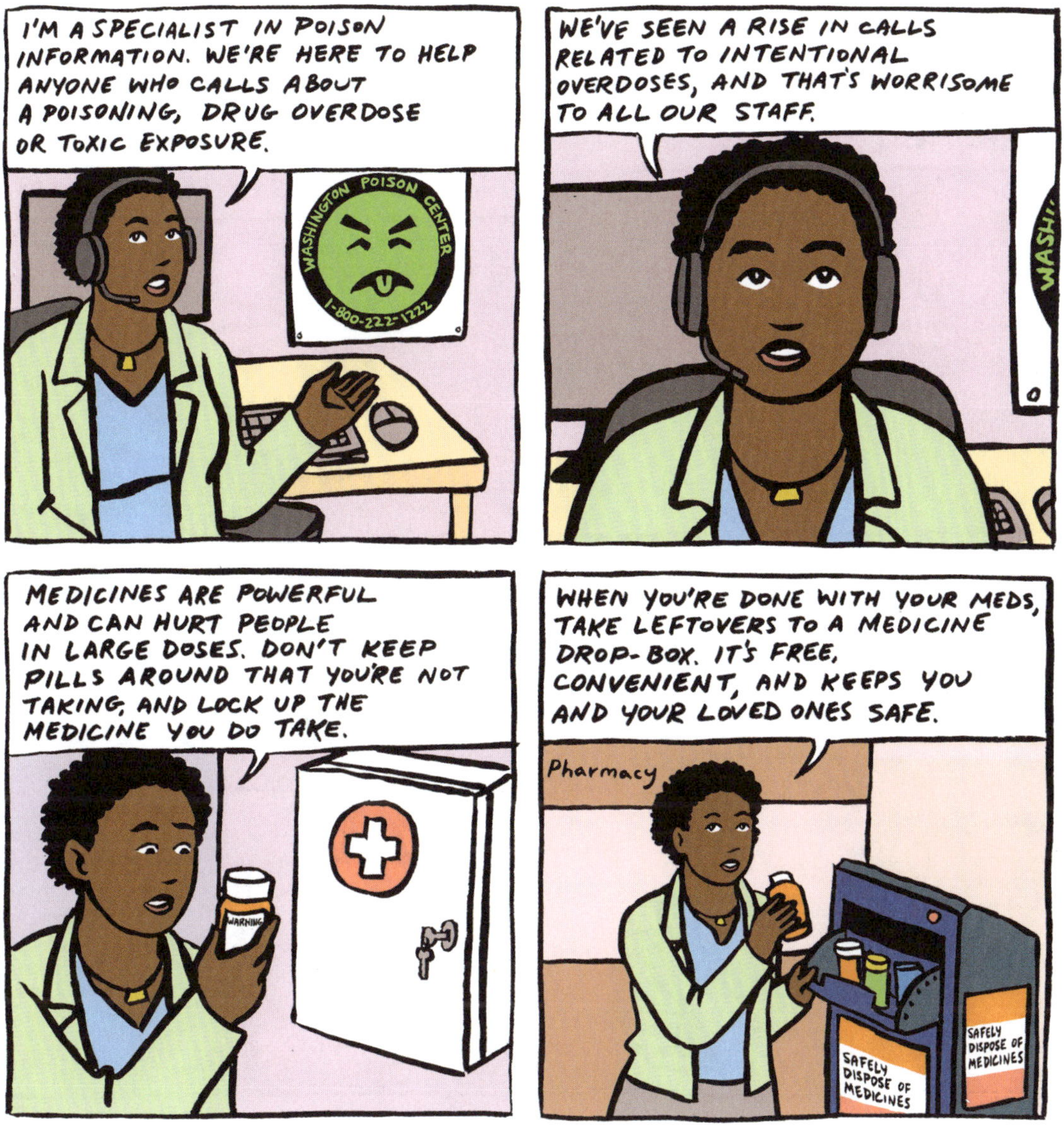
I'M A SPECIALIST IN POISON INFORMATION. WE'RE HERE TO HELP ANYONE WHO CALLS ABOUT A POISONING, DRUG OVERDOSE OR TOXIC EXPOSURE.
WASHINGTON POISON CENTER
1-800-222-1222
WE'VE SEEN A RISE IN CALLS RELATED TO INTENTIONAL OVERDOSES, AND THAT'S WORRISOME TO ALL OUR STAFF.
MEDICINES ARE POWERFUL AND CAN HURT PEOPLE IN LARGE DOSES. DON'T KEEP PILLS AROUND THAT YOU'RE NOT TAKING, AND LOCK UP THE MEDICINE YOU DO TAKE.
WARNING
WHEN YOU'RE DONE WITH YOUR MEDS, TAKE LEFTOVERS TO A MEDICINE DROP-BOX. IT'S FREE, CONVENIENT, AND KEEPS YOU AND YOUR LOVED ONES SAFE.
Pharmacy
SAFELY DISPOSE OF MEDICINES
SAFELY DISPOSE OF MEDICINES

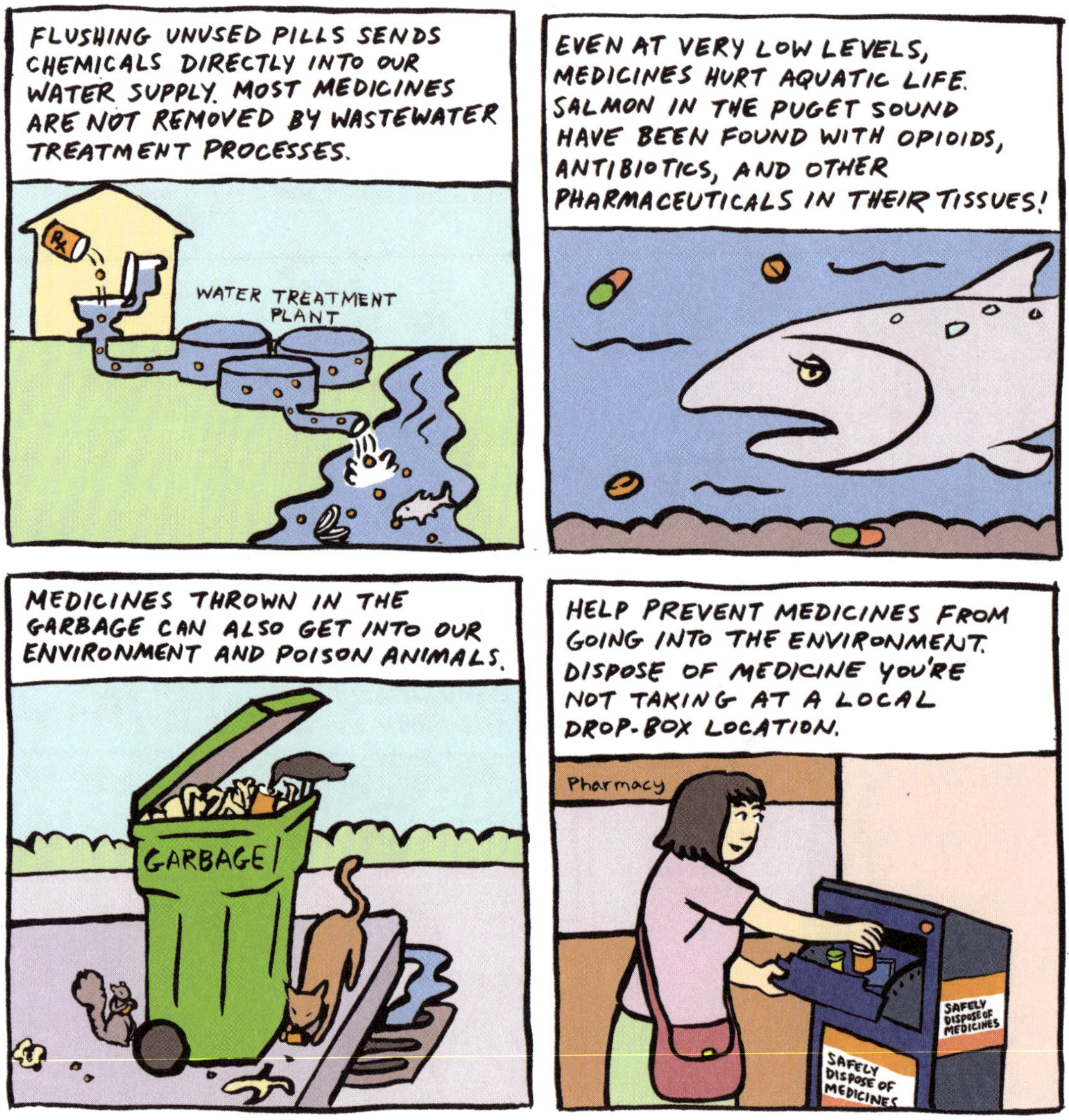
FLUSHING UNUSED PILLS SENDS CHEMICALS DIRECTLY INTO OUR WATER SUPPLY. MOST MEDICINES ARE NOT REMOVED BY WASTEWATER TREATMENT PROCESSES.
WATER TREATMENT PLANT
EVEN AT VERY LOW LEVELS, MEDICINES HURT AQUATIC LIFE. SALMON IN THE PUGET SOUND HAVE BEEN FOUND WITH OPIOIDS, ANTIBIOTICS, AND OTHER PHARMACEUTICALS IN THEIR TISSUES!
MEDICINES THROWN IN THE GARBAGE CAN ALSO GET INTO OUR ENVIRONMENT AND POISON ANIMALS.
GARBAGE
HELP PREVENT MEDICINES FROM GOING INTO THE ENVIRONMENT. DISPOSE OF MEDICINE YOU'RE NOT TAKING AT A LOCAL DROP-BOX LOCATION.
Pharmacy
SAFELY DISPOSE OF MEDICINES

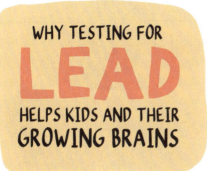

WHY TESTING FOR **LEAD** HELPS KIDS AND THEIR GROWING BRAINS

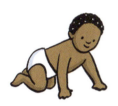
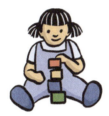
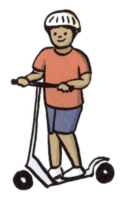
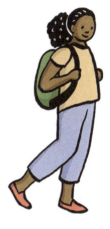

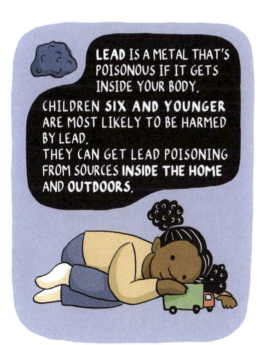

LEAD IS A METAL THAT'S POISONOUS IF IT GETS INSIDE YOUR BODY.

CHILDREN **SIX AND YOUNGER** ARE MOST LIKELY TO BE HARMED BY LEAD.

THEY CAN GET LEAD POISONING FROM SOURCES **INSIDE THE HOME** AND **OUTDOORS**.

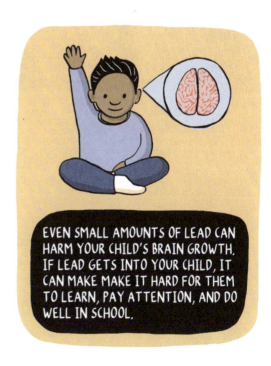

EVEN SMALL AMOUNTS OF LEAD CAN HARM YOUR CHILD'S BRAIN GROWTH. IF LEAD GETS INTO YOUR CHILD, IT CAN MAKE MAKE IT HARD FOR THEM TO LEARN, PAY ATTENTION, AND DO WELL IN SCHOOL.

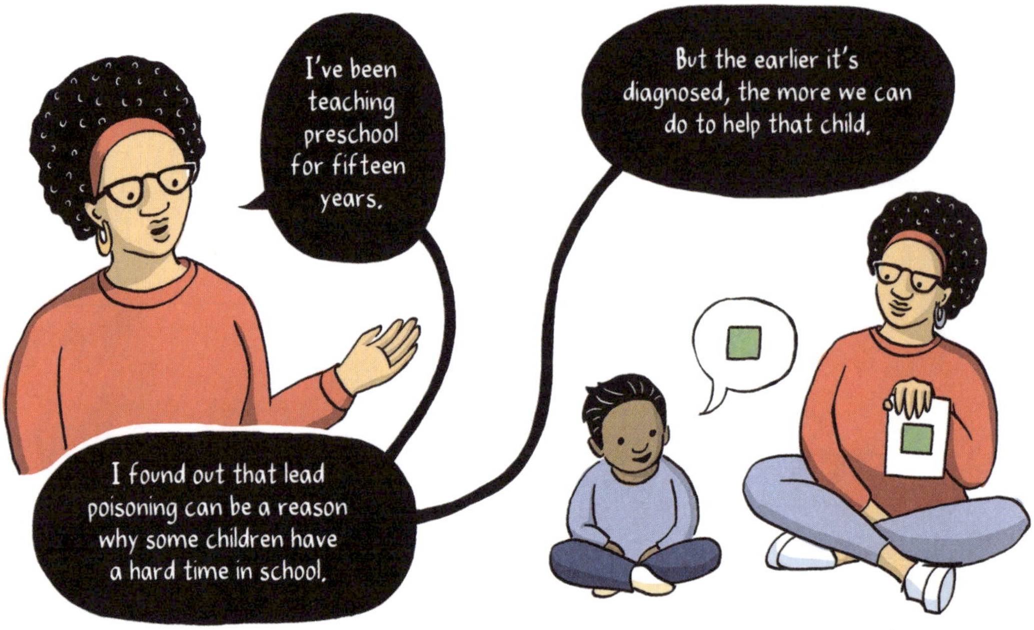
I've been teaching preschool for fifteen years.
I found out that lead poisoning can be a reason why some children have a hard time in school.
But the earlier it's diagnosed, the more we can do to help that child.

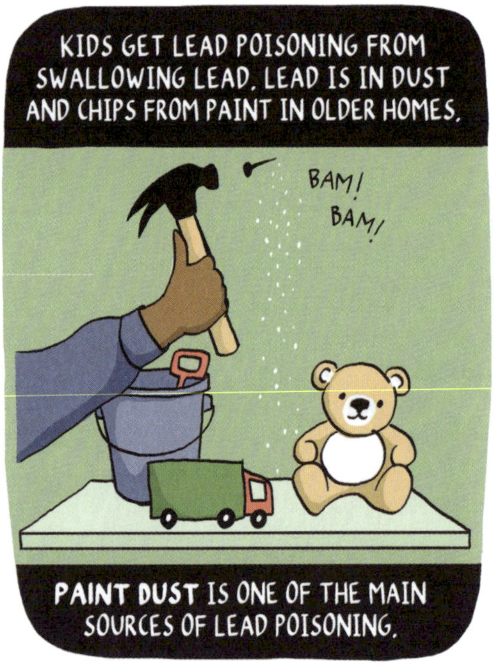
KIDS GET LEAD POISONING FROM SWALLOWING LEAD. LEAD IS IN DUST AND CHIPS FROM PAINT IN OLDER HOMES.
BAM!
BAM!
PAINT DUST IS ONE OF THE MAIN SOURCES OF LEAD POISONING.

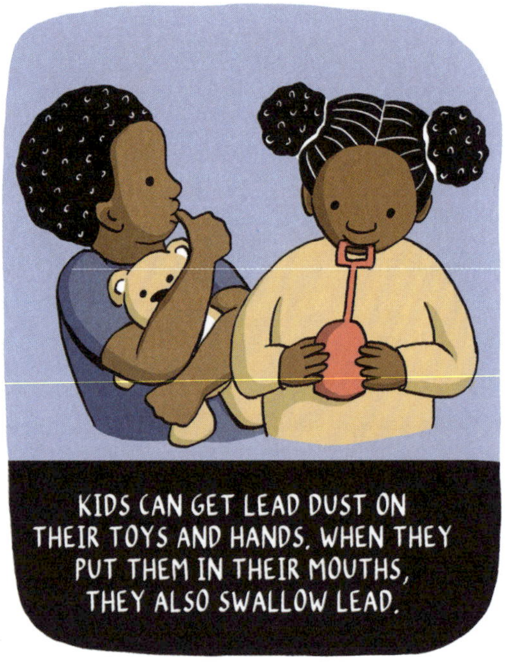
KIDS CAN GET LEAD DUST ON THEIR TOYS AND HANDS. WHEN THEY PUT THEM IN THEIR MOUTHS, THEY ALSO SWALLOW LEAD.

OTHER THINGS THAT MAY ALSO CONTAIN LEAD:

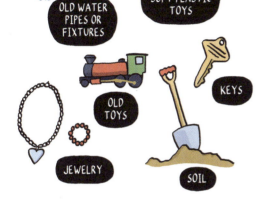

OLD WATER PIPES OR FIXTURES

INEXPENSIVE, SOFT PLASTIC TOYS

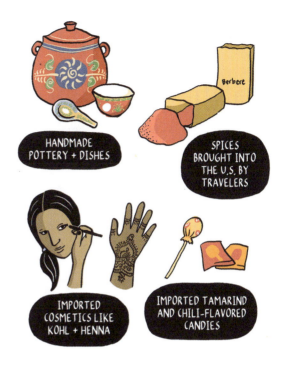

HANDMADE POTTERY + DISHES

SPICES BROUGHT INTO THE U.S. BY TRAVELERS

OLD TOYS

KEYS

JEWELRY

SOIL

IMPORTED COSMETICS LIKE KOHL + HENNA

IMPORTED TAMARIND AND CHILI-FLAVORED CANDIES

CHILDREN NEED A BLOOD LEAD SCREENING TEST IF THEY:

 SPEND TIME REGULARLY AT A HOUSE BUILT BEFORE 1950, OR ONE BUILT BEFORE 1978 THAT HAS RECENT REPAIRS OR IMPROVEMENTS.

 HAVE A LOWER FAMILY INCOME.

 HAVE A FRIEND OR SIBLING WITH ELEVATED BLOOD LEAD LEVEL.

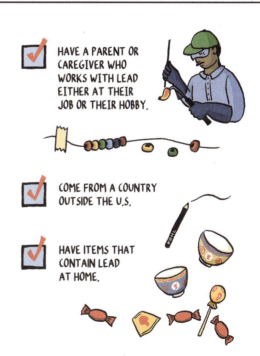 HAVE A PARENT OR CAREGIVER WHO WORKS WITH LEAD EITHER AT THEIR JOB OR THEIR HOBBY.

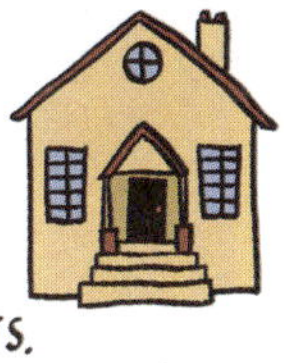

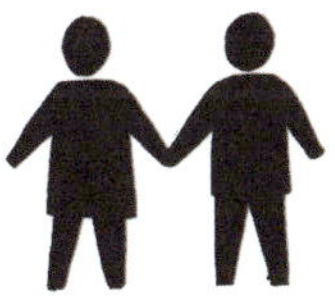

COME FROM A COUNTRY OUTSIDE THE U.S.

 HAVE ITEMS THAT CONTAIN LEAD AT HOME.

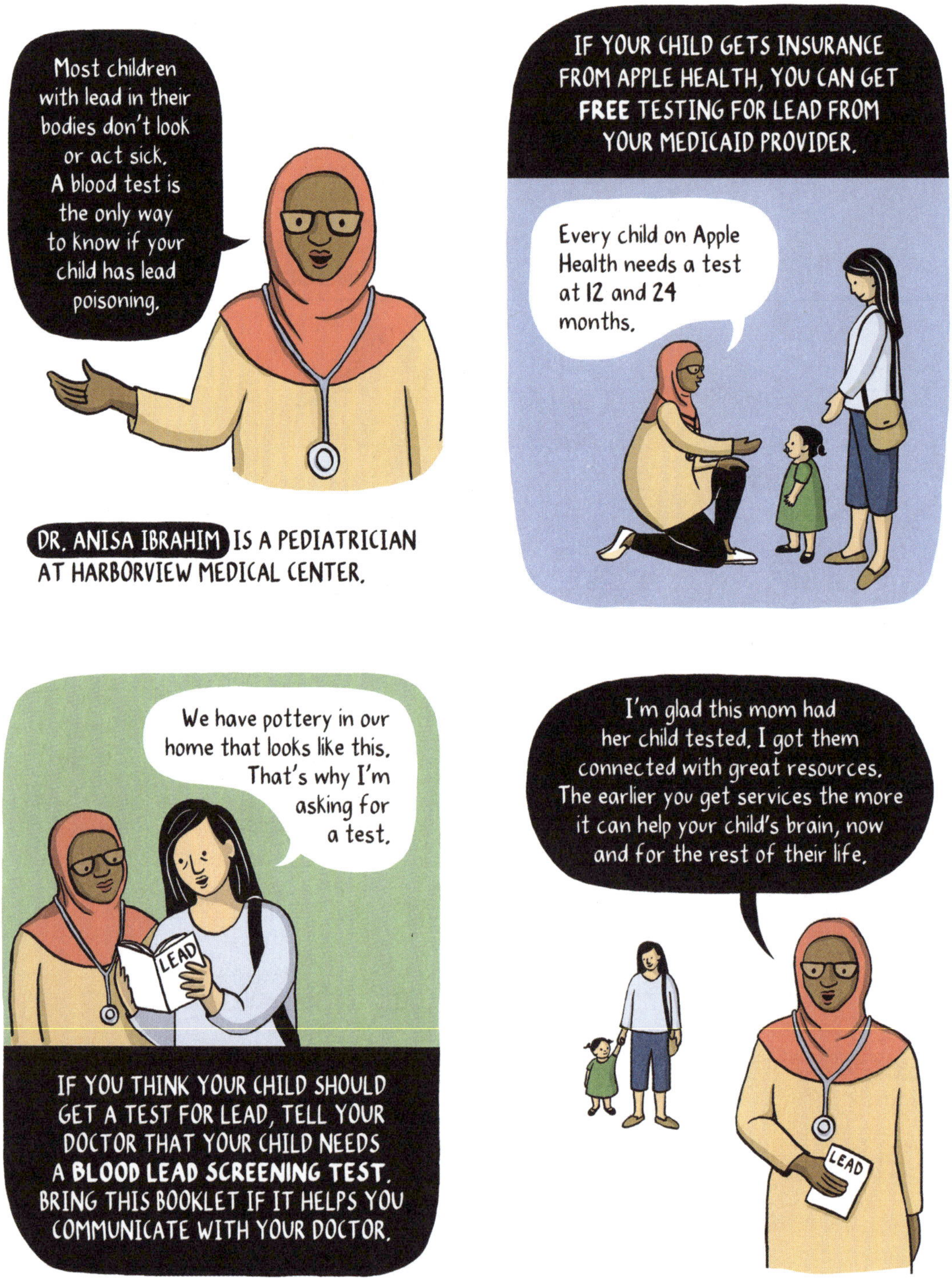
Most children with lead in their bodies don't look or act sick. A blood test is the only way to know if your child has lead poisoning.
DR. ANISA IBRAHIM IS A PEDIATRICIAN AT HARBORVIEW MEDICAL CENTER.
IF YOUR CHILD GETS INSURANCE FROM APPLE HEALTH, YOU CAN GET **FREE** TESTING FOR LEAD FROM YOUR MEDICAID PROVIDER.
Every child on Apple Health needs a test at 12 and 24 months.
We have pottery in our home that looks like this. That's why I'm asking for a test.
LEAD
IF YOU THINK YOUR CHILD SHOULD GET A TEST FOR LEAD, TELL YOUR DOCTOR THAT YOUR CHILD NEEDS A **BLOOD LEAD SCREENING TEST**. BRING THIS BOOKLET IF IT HELPS YOU COMMUNICATE WITH YOUR DOCTOR.
I'm glad this mom had her child tested. I got them connected with great resources. The earlier you get services the more it can help your child's brain, now and for the rest of their life.
LEAD

Discussion

Public health is rich in information—frequently excellent, evidence-based information—that can have a profound influence on health and well-being. However, even when the information will potentially lengthen life spans or save people and their loved ones from serious harm, health information often can't compete with the continuous barrage of more attractive messages encountered in a typical day. The onus is on health communicators to make healthy behaviors more enticing and find ways to make health promotions stand out.

Rising to the challenge, public health communications have become savvier by adopting strategies and tactics from the commercial marketing world. The expanding field of *social marketing* recognizes that health behaviors need to be pitched to the consumer like other products. By focusing on the desires and needs of specific audiences, social marketing seeks to influence behaviors that will benefit the consumer—in this case, the consumer's individual health and, often, the greater welfare of the community.

The two comics projects shown in this chapter were used as part of larger campaigns to promote the safe disposal of prescription medicines and lead poisoning testing for children. While these comics were not developed as social marketing campaigns, the approaches used overlap with many of the principles of social marketing, including audience segmentation, strategies to overcome consumer barriers, and careful consideration of how messaging is constructed and displayed. Few public health entities have big budgets for anything like the commercial advertising campaigns that corporations run. Public health communicators need creative resources that are cost effective, flexible across multiple audiences and a breadth of marketing objectives, *and* able to grab the attention of the people they're trying to reach. As a medium for promotion, comics have the adaptability, explanatory power, and mass appeal to be a valuable element in a health campaign's marketing mix.

The Don't Hang on to Meds Campaign

Marketing Medicine Return as a New Behavior

As part of the effort to prevent opioid overdoses, King County, Washington, allows the public to return unused and expired medications for disposal by pharmaceutical companies using free drop boxes. These drop boxes are in over one hundred locations, but prior to the Don't Hang on to Meds campaign, most people didn't know that the drop boxes existed or what they were for.

King County's Heroin and Prescription Opioid Addiction Task Force needed a campaign to promote the medicine return drop boxes as well as the behavior of returning medication. Returning medications has several health benefits to individuals and the community: (1) it prevents other people from taking pills from medicine cabinets, a behavior that can lead to addiction to opioids; (2) it reduces the likelihood that someone would use medications for self-harm, including suicide; (3) it prevents children and pets from getting into the medications by accident; and (4) it keeps drugs out of the water system and environment by providing an alternative to flushing medicines or throwing them away. However, the task force staff determined that most people weren't aware of the benefits and preferred to hang on to their unused pills and medicines for cost savings and convenience. Getting people to use the drop boxes would require a shift in thinking about keeping medications.

Comics That Illustrate the Costs and Benefits of Medicine Return

For the medicine return campaign, we identified four target audiences:

- parents of children and youth,
- seniors who tend to have large caches of medications,
- health care providers (many of whom were unaware of the medicine return program), and
- environmentally minded individuals.

For these groups, medicine return comes at a cost in terms of the additional effort needed to take medicines to a drop box and the cost of purchasing new medications rather than keeping unused ones. Convincing them to return their medications required the campaign to demonstrate that the benefit would be greater than the cost.

With that in mind, I wrote a comic strip for each target audience based on interviews with people who have been affected by easy access to opioid medications, including a young woman who stole medications starting at age thirteen and a call-center operator who handled overdose calls for a poison-control hotline. Paired with the tag line "Don't Hang on to Meds," the comic strips illustrate specific benefits for returning medication that align with each audience segment. For seniors, a potential benefit is to prevent accidental poisoning of a grandchild or pet; for someone who cares about the environment, it may be to keep local waters and wildlife free from contamination; for a parent, it may be to prevent youth from taking drugs for self-medication or intentional overdose.

Another key barrier to medicine return was that people didn't know where to return their medications. The medicine drop boxes look very similar to mailboxes and often escape notice (perhaps by design, as they were installed by the pharmaceutical companies who are required to pay for the disposal). For the Don't Hang on to Meds campaign, the comic panels prominently featured images of the drop boxes in pharmacy settings so that audiences would know where to find them.

Later I took pills from other medicine cabinets.
DON'T HANG ON TO MEDS
Find a drop-box near you!
MedicineReturn.org
I was a good kid.
DON'T HANG ON TO MEDS
International District/Chinatown
FIND A MEDICINE RETURN DROP-BOX

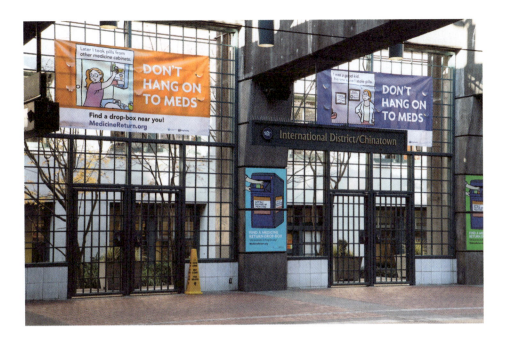

Fig. 3.1. The sequenced panels for the *Don't Hang on to Meds* comics were made into large-scale banners that could be read along a mass transit platform. Artwork by Tatiana Gill. Photo: Meredith Li-Vollmer.

The Look and Feel of the *Don't Hang on to Meds* Comics

Using the scripts, artist Tatiana Gill drew four- to six-panel comics with relatable characters as the narrators. Tatiana's drawings have a friendly appeal, with confident lines, simple yet expressive faces, and a strong color sense. They also have a spontaneity that makes the cartoon characters feel like real people and lends an authenticity to the stories. An effort was also made to represent people from different racial and ethnic groups, reflecting the people who live in King County, and to demonstrate how access to opioid medication affects people from across these groups.

Making *Don't Hang on to Meds* Visible

The *Don't Hang on to Meds* comics could be adapted to multiple formats, which made it easy to place them directly in the path of consumers. To get the campaign in front of target audiences, we promoted the comics as:

- posts on Facebook, Instagram, and Twitter, using square panels and limiting the length of each comic to four to six panels (and we boosted the posts to reach the target demographics, e.g., parents of young children, older adults, people with interests in environmental issues);

- print materials, including postcards for health care providers to give to patients, posters for display at pharmacies and other drop box locations, and printed bags for pharmacies to use;
- entries on the health department's blog;
- interior and exterior bus signage, with shortened versions of the comics to make it easy to read them at a glance; and
- promotional materials hung inside transit stations, covering two downtown Seattle transit stations with giant campaign posters and banners on interior walls and platforms (fig. 3.1).

Comics for a Lead Testing Campaign

Promoting Lead Testing for Children

Another health promotion comics campaign sought to raise awareness of household exposure to lead and increase the number of young children tested for lead poisoning. Household exposure to lead is commonplace, especially in older affordable housing, and it's most harmful to children, whose brains are still developing. The lead and toxics program at Public Health—Seattle & King County requested a campaign to encourage parents to ask their health care providers to test their children for lead; the target audiences were families of toddlers and preschoolers in neighborhoods with older housing, where lead exposure is more common, and in specific immigrant communities, whose households are more likely to have imported products containing lead. With early enough detection of lead poisoning, social workers and educators can provide therapies to counter developmental impacts of lead exposure.

Barriers to Getting Children Tested

One of the challenges in reaching the audience is that lead poisoning is an off-putting topic that presents psychological and emotional barriers. Some parents may have a hard time accepting that something as harmful as lead could be in the safe environment of their own homes. A lack of self-efficacy may influence some to tune out messages if they feel like there's nothing they can do for a child who has already been exposed to lead; from this perspective, the fear of receiving a positive test for lead poisoning would make testing undesirable. Other parents may not feel comfortable asking a doctor for a lead test and may find it even more difficult to press for a test if the health care provider is not aware of lead testing guidance and doesn't see the need.

The Comic: *Why Testing for Lead Helps Kids and Their Growing Brains*

As the centerpiece of the campaign, the comic *Why Testing for Lead Helps Kids and Their Growing Brains* emphasizes the positive benefits of lead testing to counter the alarm raised by the possibility of lead poisoning. The comic features the voices of experts who are credible to parents—a preschool teacher and a well-respected local pediatrician. These characters explain how lead can harm children's learning and development, but to prevent parents from feeling helpless, they also provide encouraging words about the availability of support services and the advantages of early detection.

Staff who worked in the target communities reported that many parents felt uncomfortable asking their doctors for a lead test because of the deference they felt toward medical providers. They also found that some health care professionals were unaware of the risks of lead and didn't see a need for testing, even when parents asked for a test. With this input in mind, *Why Testing for Lead Helps Kids and Their Growing Brains* took the form of a mini-comic book that parents could take to their medical appointments. The expository text encourages parents to show the comic book to the clinician to assist with communication (fig. 3.2). The parent in the illustration also models the desired behavior of asking for a test. In this way, the comic book can be used as a physical tool for parents to advocate for their children, in addition to promoting the specific behavior.

We have pottery in our home that looks like this. That's why I'm asking for a test.
LEAD
IF YOU THINK YOUR CHILD SHOULD GET A TEST FOR LEAD, TELL YOUR DOCTOR THAT YOUR CHILD NEEDS A BLOOD LEAD SCREENING TEST. BRING THIS BOOKLET IF IT HELPS YOU COMMUNICATE WITH YOUR DOCTOR.
13

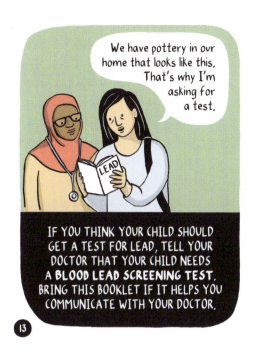

Fig. 3.2. This panel demonstrates to parents how they can physically use the mini-comic book as a tool to communicate with their child's health care provider. We added this to the comic after hearing that some parents needed a way to advocate for lead testing. Artwork by Amy Camber for *Why Testing for Lead Helps Kids and Their Growing Brains.* Courtesy of Public Health—Seattle & King County.

Artist Amy Camber's clean line work, color selection, deft placement of text, and skill in depicting warm images of diverse families are also instrumental to the promotional strategy. Her charming illustrations of tots in preschool settings connote feelings of caring, reinforce the positive messages, and are visually inviting. The color palette—reminiscent of toy blocks in soft shades of blue, green, red, and golden yellow—signals to parents of young children that the information is for them.

It was critical to reach parents in the immigrant communities that have higher exposure to lead. Camber crafted the illustrations using reference photos of community members and included drawings of lead-containing household objects common in the target communities, such as Chinese ceramic bowls and imported cosmetics. One of the main characters is a trusted local pediatrician who works with immigrant families.

To make sure the information was culturally relevant and actionable, members of the target communities also reviewed the script, which was translated into their languages.

Getting the Comic in the Hands of Parents

Why Lead Testing Helps Kids and Their Growing Brains was printed as an appealing, palm-sized mini-comic booklet. A miniature book invites people to pick it up and peruse it, and using high-quality photocopying on standard copier paper made it less expensive than traditional comic book printing. To put them in the hands of parents, we distributed the mini-comics to community organizations, preschools, daycare providers, and health clinics for their waiting rooms. Pages from the comic were developed into ads in ethnic print media and also as boosted content on social media targeted at parents in affected neighborhoods. The comic was also adapted into a short animated video so that voice-overs could be done in the languages of people who rely primarily on oral communication, particularly in the Somali, Khmer, and Pacific Islander communities.

Comics in the Health Promotion and Social Marketing Mix

In today's dense landscape of niche media and competition for the public's attention, public health needs every advantage to promote behaviors like asking for a lead test for your child or taking your medications to a drop box. Comics have promise as an addition to the social marketing toolbox. Highly flexible, they deliver messages that can be customized to meet a specific audience's communication needs.

Comics have the visual power to break through the clutter of competing messages. Their design and style can be tailored to specific audience segments using a myriad of stylistic choices available for comics. Mainstream comic book styles that resemble Marvel or DC comics may have appeal to particular audiences, like preteens. The CDC, among other organizations, has used this style in the *Junior Disease Detectives* comic book.[1] But many styles of comics have been relatively untapped for health promotion campaigns. For example, the grittiness and "weirdo" quality of underground "comix" may speak to certain youth subcultures; Japanese manga-style comics could attract the adolescent girls who make up a sizeable part of the manga fan base; and beautiful art comics (like Mita Mahato's *Climate Changes Health*, shown in chapter 1) may appeal to people who don't even identify as comics fans.

Comics are easily incorporated into eye-grabbing campaigns across different types of collateral material, making them a great vehicle for health promotion messages that meet the information-seeking behaviors and preferences of specific audiences. Comics adapt readily to social media, billboards, postcards, posters, flyers, ads in print publications and ethnic media, and, of course, comic books.

Finally, comics have explanatory power through storytelling and exposition that can highlight, demonstrate, and comment upon the benefits of healthy behaviors. Bite-sized stories and personal testimonies in comics form can make the pitch in economical fashion. Using comics, subject matter experts in public health can shift from thinking about promoting "facts" to developing narratives that make health promotions fit into the context of people's lives and concerns. Like other forms of advertising, comics can produce an emotional reaction that will make the marketing of healthy behaviors more persuasive, more memorable, and more resonant. Narrative comics can engage readers in the situations shown in the comic and perhaps also encourage them to consider the parts of the story that are implied but not directly shown, such as the pain a parent might feel in discovering that his child has been getting into medications in the home, or the frustrations of a child in school who has suffered from lead poisoning.

The comics I have included for this chapter have not had the benefit of the in-depth evaluation that is fundamental to a true social marketing approach. Although we have done formative evaluation for comics with members of target audiences, the limited funding and especially limited staff available to do formal evaluations in the fast pace of our health department have impeded our ability to gather data to help assess the comics' impact. The formative evaluation for *Why Testing for Lead Helps Kids and Their Growing Brains* came from reviewers in the target communities who reported that they found the comic appealing and left with better understanding of the importance of lead testing. The mini-comic also was well received by community organizations that requested copies. After the launch of the Don't Hang on to Meds comics campaign, the annual visits to the program website increased 221 percent from the year prior; however, we don't know how much of that increase can be attributed to exposure to the comics. Like many health communications efforts, it is difficult to parse the impact of these comics on behavior change, which is subject to so many social and environmental influences.

Obviously, there is need for more evaluation of comics for health promotion, including the comics that I have helped produce. As health behavior changes are difficult to attribute directly to exposure to health communications, qualitative evaluations that focus on consumers' reactions and readings of health promotion comics could be particularly illuminating. This type of evaluation could direct health communicators to possibilities for comics to spark a deeper level of engagement in health promotion materials.

4.

Comics for Advocacy and Activism

The Comics

Selections from *Sketches Outside the Margins: Patient Stories from the Seattle / King County Clinic* (2016–18), edited by Meredith Li-Vollmer

121 "Felipe," by Tatiana Gill, 2018. Courtesy of Seattle / King County Clinic.

122 "Mixed Blessing," by Meredith Li-Vollmer, 2017. Courtesy of Seattle / King County Clinic.

123 "Imagine," by Kelly Froh, 2017. Courtesy of Seattle / King County Clinic.

124 "Ashley," by David Lasky, 2017. Courtesy of Seattle / King County Clinic.

125 "Mike Archer," by Ellen Forney, 2018. Courtesy of Seattle / King County Clinic.

126 "Lolinda," by Amy Camber, 2018. Courtesy of Seattle / King County Clinic.

127 "Health Fair," by Meredith Li-Vollmer, 2018. Courtesy of Seattle / King County Clinic.

128 "Puppy Love," by Roberta Gregory, 2018. Courtesy of Seattle / King County Clinic.

129 "Catching Up," by Meredith Li-Vollmer, 2018. Courtesy of Seattle / King County Clinic.

130 "For Janet," written by Meredith Li-Vollmer, artwork by David Lasky, 2018. Courtesy of Seattle / King County Clinic.

134 "Epilogue," by Meredith Li-Vollmer, 2018. Courtesy of Seattle / King County Clinic.

Selections from *Comics 4 Health Coverage: Why Health Insurance Matters in Four Panels* (2013), edited by Meredith Li-Vollmer

139 "Lumps," by Kelly Froh, 2013.

140 Untitled comic by David Lasky, 2013.

141 "Care," by Mita Mahato, 2013.

142 "Only in America," by Roberta Gregory, 2013.

Selections from *Lines Drawn: Parents and Teachers Who've Had Enough* (2018), edited by Meredith Li-Vollmer and Mita Mahato

143 "Window," by Mita Mahato, 2018.

144 "False Choice," by Meredith Li-Vollmer, 2018.

145 "Drilled," by Ellen Forney, 2018.

147 Untitled comic by Rachel Scheer, 2018.

148 "Climate Change," written by Adam Bessie, artwork by Marc Parenteau, 2018.

Comics About a Local Health Department

150 "Stretched Thin: An Outbreak Story," by Meredith Li-Vollmer, 2017. Courtesy of Public Health—Seattle & King County.

153 Excerpt from *The Public Health Notebook*, by Meredith Li-Vollmer, 2019. Courtesy of Public Health—Seattle & King County.

ALL PEOPLE SHOULD HAVE ACCESS TO HEALTHCARE AS A RIGHT, JUST AS PUBLIC EDUCATION THROUGH HIGH SCHOOL.
DELORES KANNAS (VOLUNTEER)
I SAW PEOPLE THAT WERE JUST ELATED TO HAVE SOME DENTAL WORK DONE.
ONE GIRL IN PARTICULAR...SHE HAD A TOOTH REPLACED WHERE SHE WAS MISSING A TOOTH IN THE FRONT. TOTALLY DIFFERENT PERSON. IT WAS LIKE SHE WON THE LOTTERY.
TONY MARINICH (PATIENT)
THE SEATTLE/KING COUNTY CLINIC (SKCC) IS A FREE POP-UP CLINIC.
IN 2016 IT OFFERED DENTAL, VISION, AND MEDICAL CARE TO 4,492 PEOPLE OVER FOUR DAYS AT KEY ARENA.
WITH THE AFFORDABLE CARE ACT (ACA) THE UNINSURED RATE HAS FALLEN FROM 15.7% TO 8.6% IN 2016.
UNINSURED
296.5M
27.9M
31M
INSURED
UNDERINSURED
BUT MANY NEED MORE INSURANCE.
POP-UPS GIVE TEMPORARY RELIEF TO RURAL AND URBAN COMMUNITIES OPERATING IN A FRACTURED HEALTHCARE SYSTEM.
IT'S A GRASSROOTS EFFORT PUT ON WITHOUT FEDERAL FUNDING BY 115 ORGANIZATIONS AND STAFFED ALMOST ENTIRELY BY THEIR 3,947 VOLUNTEERS.
I LOOK AT HEALTH CARE ACCESS AS A QUILT AND IT'S JUST ONE MORE PATCH.
MEDICARE
MEDICAID
SKCC
CRITICAL ACCESS HOSPITALS
CHRISTINE LINDQUIST
EXECUTIVE DIRECTOR
WASHINGTON HEALTHCARE ACCESS ALLIANCE
ADULT DENTAL NOW IS COVERED BY MEDICAID [IN WASHINGTON].
THIS IS RARE.
BUT IF YOU DON'T HAVE SOMEONE WHO CAN GIVE YOU THE CARE IT DOESN'T REALLY MATTER.
DENTIST
ØRESULTS

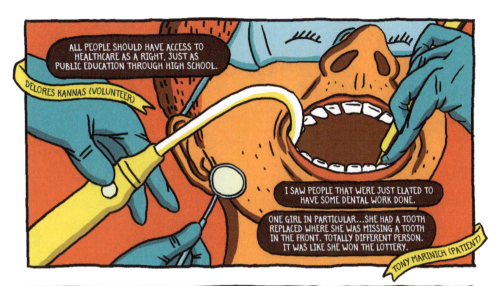

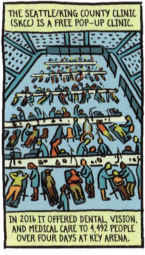

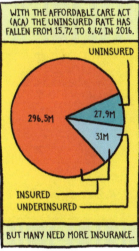

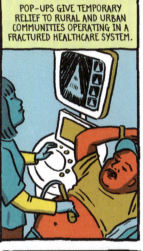

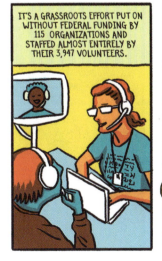

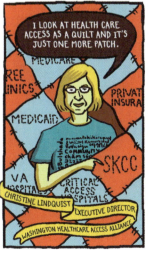

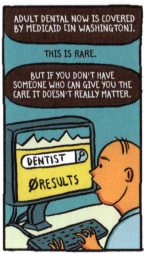

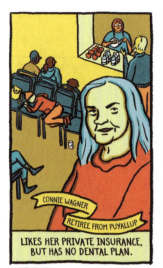

CONNIE WAGNER
RETIREE FROM PUYALLUP

LIKES HER PRIVATE INSURANCE, BUT HAS NO DENTAL PLAN.

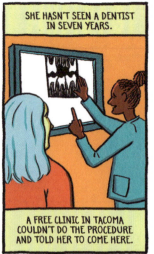

SHE HASN'T SEEN A DENTIST IN SEVEN YEARS.

A FREE CLINIC IN TACOMA COULDN'T DO THE PROCEDURE AND TOLD HER TO COME HERE.

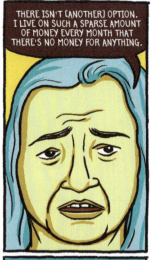

THERE ISN'T [ANOTHER] OPTION. I LIVE ON SUCH A SPARSE AMOUNT OF MONEY EVERY MONTH THAT THERE'S NO MONEY FOR ANYTHING.

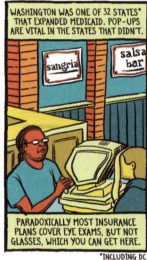

WASHINGTON WAS ONE OF 32 STATES* THAT EXPANDED MEDICAID. POP-UPS ARE VITAL IN THE STATES THAT DIDN'T.

PARADOXICALLY MOST INSURANCE PLANS COVER EYE EXAMS, BUT NOT GLASSES, WHICH YOU CAN GET HERE.

*INCLUDING DC

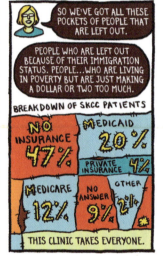

SO WE'VE GOT ALL THESE POCKETS OF PEOPLE THAT ARE LEFT OUT.

PEOPLE WHO ARE LEFT OUT BECAUSE OF THEIR IMMIGRATION STATUS. PEOPLE...WHO ARE LIVING IN POVERTY BUT ARE JUST MAKING A DOLLAR OR TWO TOO MUCH.

BREAKDOWN OF SKCC PATIENTS

NO INSURANCE 47%
MEDICAID 20%
PRIVATE INSURANCE 4%
MEDICARE 12%
NO ANSWER 9%
OTHER 2%

THIS CLINIC TAKES EVERYONE.

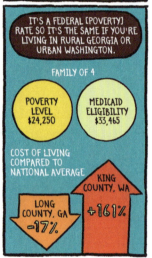

IT'S A FEDERAL [POVERTY] RATE SO IT'S THE SAME IF YOU'RE LIVING IN RURAL GEORGIA OR URBAN WASHINGTON.

FAMILY OF 4

POVERTY LEVEL $24,250

MEDICAID ELIGIBILITY $33,465

COST OF LIVING COMPARED TO NATIONAL AVERAGE

LONG COUNTY, GA -17%

KING COUNTY, WA +161%

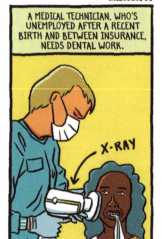

A MEDICAL TECHNICIAN, WHO'S UNEMPLOYED AFTER A RECENT BIRTH AND BETWEEN INSURANCE, NEEDS DENTAL WORK.

X-RAY

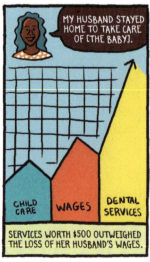

MY HUSBAND STAYED HOME TO TAKE CARE OF [THE BABY].

CHILD CARE
WAGES
DENTAL SERVICES

SERVICES WORTH $500 OUTWEIGHED THE LOSS OF HER HUSBAND'S WAGES.

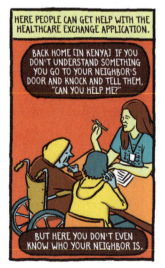

HERE PEOPLE CAN GET HELP WITH THE HEALTHCARE EXCHANGE APPLICATION.

BACK HOME [IN KENYA] IF YOU DON'T UNDERSTAND SOMETHING YOU GO TO YOUR NEIGHBOR'S DOOR AND KNOCK AND TELL THEM, "CAN YOU HELP ME?"

BUT HERE YOU DON'T EVEN KNOW WHO YOUR NEIGHBOR IS.

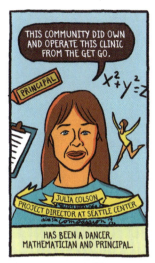

THIS COMMUNITY DID OWN AND OPERATE THIS CLINIC FROM THE GET GO.

PRINCIPAL

$x^2 + y^2 = z$

JULIA COLSON
PROJECT DIRECTOR AT SEATTLE CENTER

HAS BEEN A DANCER, MATHEMATICIAN AND PRINCIPAL.

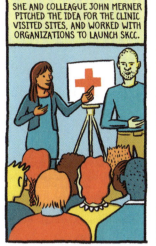

SHE AND COLLEAGUE JOHN MERNER PITCHED THE IDEA FOR THE CLINIC VISITED SITES, AND WORKED WITH ORGANIZATIONS TO LAUNCH SKCC.

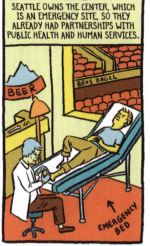

SEATTLE OWNS THE CENTER, WHICH IS AN EMERGENCY SITE, SO THEY ALREADY HAD PARTNERSHIPS WITH PUBLIC HEALTH AND HUMAN SERVICES.

BEER

BROS BAGEL

EMERGENCY BED

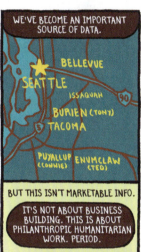

WE'VE BECOME AN IMPORTANT SOURCE OF DATA.

BELLEVUE

SEATTLE

ISSAQUAH 90

BURIEN (TONY)

TACOMA

PUYALLUP (CONNIE) ENUMCLAW (TED)

BUT THIS ISN'T MARKETABLE INFO.

IT'S NOT ABOUT BUSINESS BUILDING. THIS IS ABOUT PHILANTHROPIC HUMANITARIAN WORK. PERIOD.

*PATIENTS CAME FROM 262 ZIPCODES

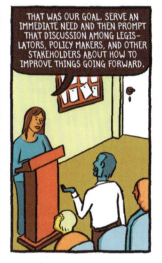

THAT WAS OUR GOAL. SERVE AN IMMEDIATE NEED AND THEN PROMPT THAT DISCUSSION AMONG LEGISLATORS, POLICY MAKERS, AND OTHER STAKEHOLDERS ABOUT HOW TO IMPROVE THINGS GOING FORWARD.

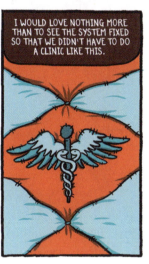

I WOULD LOVE NOTHING MORE THAN TO SEE THE SYSTEM FIXED SO THAT WE DIDN'T HAVE TO DO A CLINIC LIKE THIS.

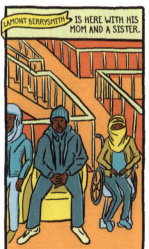

LAMONT BERRYSMITH IS HERE WITH HIS MOM AND A SISTER.

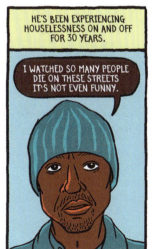

HE'S BEEN EXPERIENCING HOUSELESSNESS ON AND OFF FOR 30 YEARS.

I WATCHED SO MANY PEOPLE DIE ON THESE STREETS IT'S NOT EVEN FUNNY.

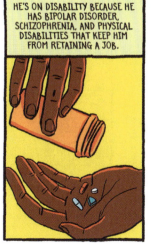

HE'S ON DISABILITY BECAUSE HE HAS BIPOLAR DISORDER, SCHIZOPHRENIA, AND PHYSICAL DISABILITIES THAT KEEP HIM FROM RETAINING A JOB.

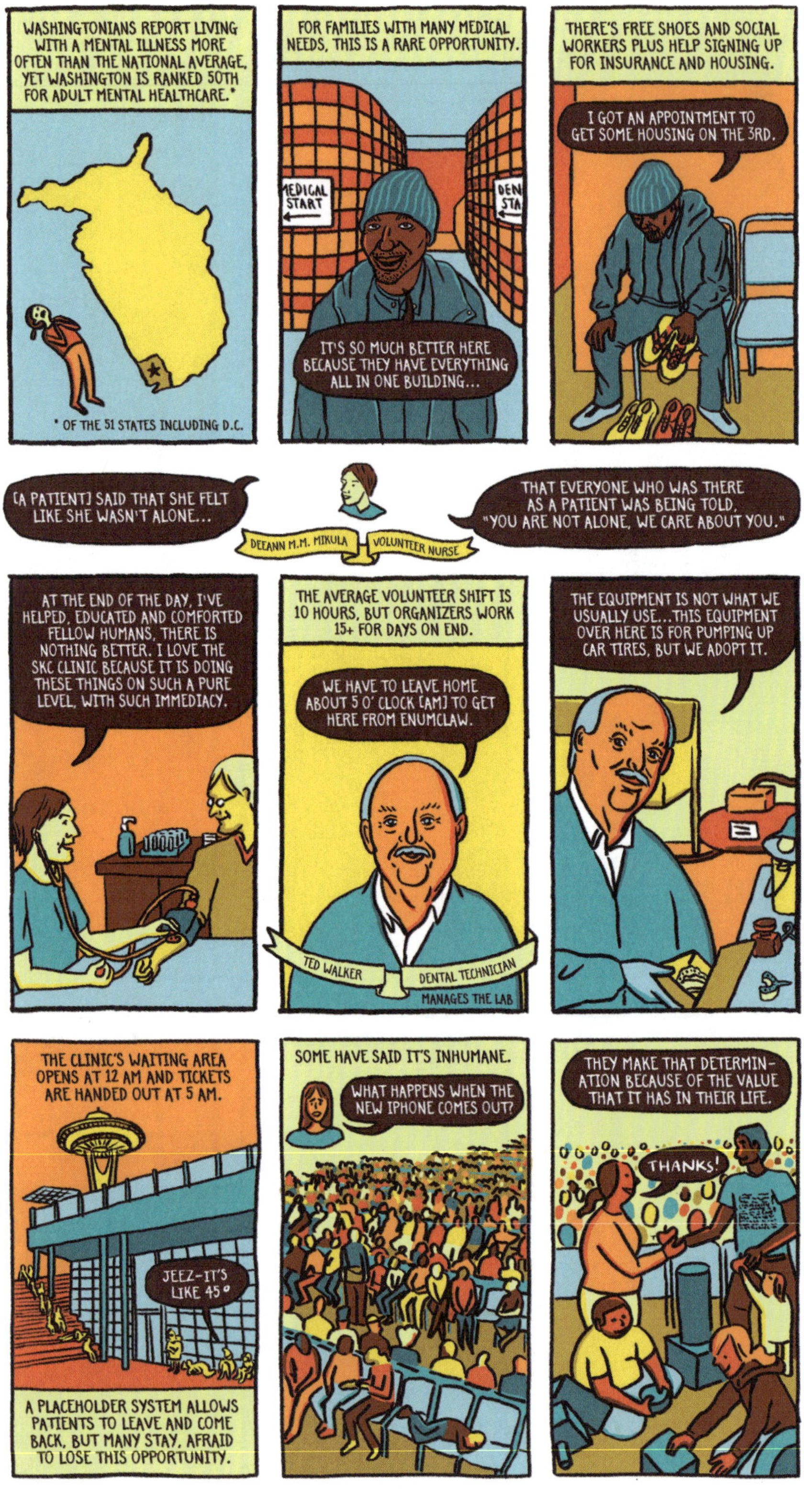

WASHINGTONIANS REPORT LIVING WITH A MENTAL ILLNESS MORE OFTEN THAN THE NATIONAL AVERAGE, YET WASHINGTON IS RANKED 50TH FOR ADULT MENTAL HEALTHCARE.*
* OF THE 51 STATES INCLUDING D.C.
FOR FAMILIES WITH MANY MEDICAL NEEDS, THIS IS A RARE OPPORTUNITY.
IT'S SO MUCH BETTER HERE BECAUSE THEY HAVE EVERYTHING ALL IN ONE BUILDING...
THERE'S FREE SHOES AND SOCIAL WORKERS PLUS HELP SIGNING UP FOR INSURANCE AND HOUSING.
I GOT AN APPOINTMENT TO GET SOME HOUSING ON THE 3RD.
[A PATIENT] SAID THAT SHE FELT LIKE SHE WASN'T ALONE...
DEEANN M.M. MIKULA
VOLUNTEER NURSE
THAT EVERYONE WHO WAS THERE AS A PATIENT WAS BEING TOLD, "YOU ARE NOT ALONE, WE CARE ABOUT YOU."
AT THE END OF THE DAY, I'VE HELPED, EDUCATED AND COMFORTED FELLOW HUMANS, THERE IS NOTHING BETTER. I LOVE THE SKC CLINIC BECAUSE IT IS DOING THESE THINGS ON SUCH A PURE LEVEL, WITH SUCH IMMEDIACY.
THE AVERAGE VOLUNTEER SHIFT IS 10 HOURS, BUT ORGANIZERS WORK 15+ FOR DAYS ON END.
WE HAVE TO LEAVE HOME ABOUT 5 O' CLOCK [AM] TO GET HERE FROM ENUMCLAW.
TED WALKER
DENTAL TECHNICIAN
MANAGES THE LAB
THE EQUIPMENT IS NOT WHAT WE USUALLY USE...THIS EQUIPMENT OVER HERE IS FOR PUMPING UP CAR TIRES, BUT WE ADOPT IT.
THE CLINIC'S WAITING AREA OPENS AT 12 AM AND TICKETS ARE HANDED OUT AT 5 AM.
JEEZ–IT'S LIKE 45°
A PLACEHOLDER SYSTEM ALLOWS PATIENTS TO LEAVE AND COME BACK, BUT MANY STAY, AFRAID TO LOSE THIS OPPORTUNITY.
SOME HAVE SAID IT'S INHUMANE.
WHAT HAPPENS WHEN THE NEW IPHONE COMES OUT?
THEY MAKE THAT DETERMINATION BECAUSE OF THE VALUE THAT IT HAS IN THEIR LIFE.
THANKS!

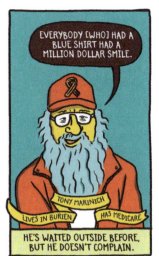

EVERYBODY [WHO] HAD A BLUE SHIRT HAD A MILLION DOLLAR SMILE.

TONY MARINICH
LIVES IN BURIEN · HAS MEDICARE

HE'S WAITED OUTSIDE BEFORE, BUT HE DOESN'T COMPLAIN.

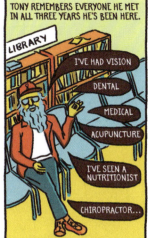

TONY REMEMBERS EVERYONE HE MET IN ALL THREE YEARS HE'S BEEN HERE.

LIBRARY

I'VE HAD VISION
DENTAL
MEDICAL
ACUPUNCTURE
I'VE SEEN A NUTRITIONIST
CHIROPRACTOR...

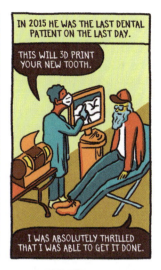

IN 2015 HE WAS THE LAST DENTAL PATIENT ON THE LAST DAY.

THIS WILL 3D PRINT YOUR NEW TOOTH.

I WAS ABSOLUTELY THRILLED THAT I WAS ABLE TO GET IT DONE.

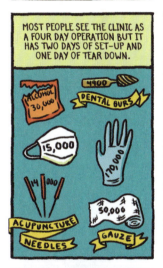

MOST PEOPLE SEE THE CLINIC AS A FOUR DAY OPERATION BUT IT HAS TWO DAYS OF SET-UP AND ONE DAY OF TEAR DOWN.

ALCOHOL 30,000
4900 DENTAL BURS
15,000
170,000
14,000
50,000
ACUPUNCTURE NEEDLES
GAUZE

THEN THERE'S MONTHS OF FOLLOWING UP:

ORDERING AND INVENTORYING SUPPLIES, SCANNING, PROCESSING, AND STORING RECORDS FOR 4,492 PATIENTS, PROCESSING 2,600 LABS, SENDING OUT REFERRALS, RECRUITING AND REGISTERING VOLUNTEERS, CHECKING LICENSES AND MALPRACTICE INSURANCE FOR HEALTHCARE PROFESSIONALS, FUNDRAISING, DISTRIBUTING 1,200 GLASSES, SECURING IN-KIND DONATIONS, CREATING AND DISTRIBUTING HEALTHCARE AND REGISTRATION FORMS, ORIENTATION, AND INFO MATERIALS, SIGNS, ADS, MAPS, AND PRESS RELEASES, COLLECTING AND INTERPRETING DATA, PATIENT OUTREACH IN MULTIPLE LANGUAGES, BIOHAZARD WASTE DISPOSAL, INTEGRATION AND OPERATIONS OF SERVICE PROVIDERS (DENTAL EQUIPMENT, DENTAL STERILIZATION, VISION EQUIPMENT, DENTAL X-RAYS, MEDICAL X-RAYS, ULTRASOUND, EKG, MEDICAL LAB, DENTAL LAB, SECURE DOCUMENT RETENTION AND SHREDDING, REMOTE INTERPRETATION SYSTEM, DENTAL VANS, MAMMOGRAPHY VAN, ETC.) PLANNING, ORDERING, AND FEEDING VOLUNTEERS AND PATIENTS, REPORTING CASES OF POSITIVE INFECTIOUS DISEASES TO PUBLIC HEALTH PER THE LAW...

IT IS FAR FROM OVER.

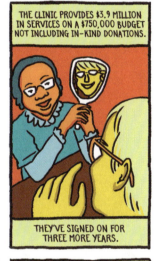

THE CLINIC PROVIDES $3.9 MILLION IN SERVICES ON A $750,000 BUDGET NOT INCLUDING IN-KIND DONATIONS.

THEY'VE SIGNED ON FOR THREE MORE YEARS.

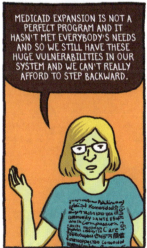

MEDICAID EXPANSION IS NOT A PERFECT PROGRAM AND IT HASN'T MET EVERYBODY'S NEEDS AND SO WE STILL HAVE THESE HUGE VULNERABILITIES IN OUR SYSTEM AND WE CAN'T REALLY AFFORD TO STEP BACKWARD.

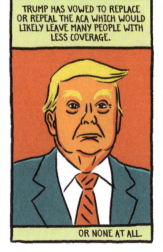

TRUMP HAS VOWED TO REPLACE OR REPEAL THE ACA WHICH WOULD LIKELY LEAVE MANY PEOPLE WITH LESS COVERAGE.

OR NONE AT ALL.

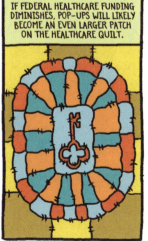

IF FEDERAL HEALTHCARE FUNDING DIMINISHES, POP-UPS WILL LIKELY BECOME AN EVEN LARGER PATCH ON THE HEALTHCARE QUILT.

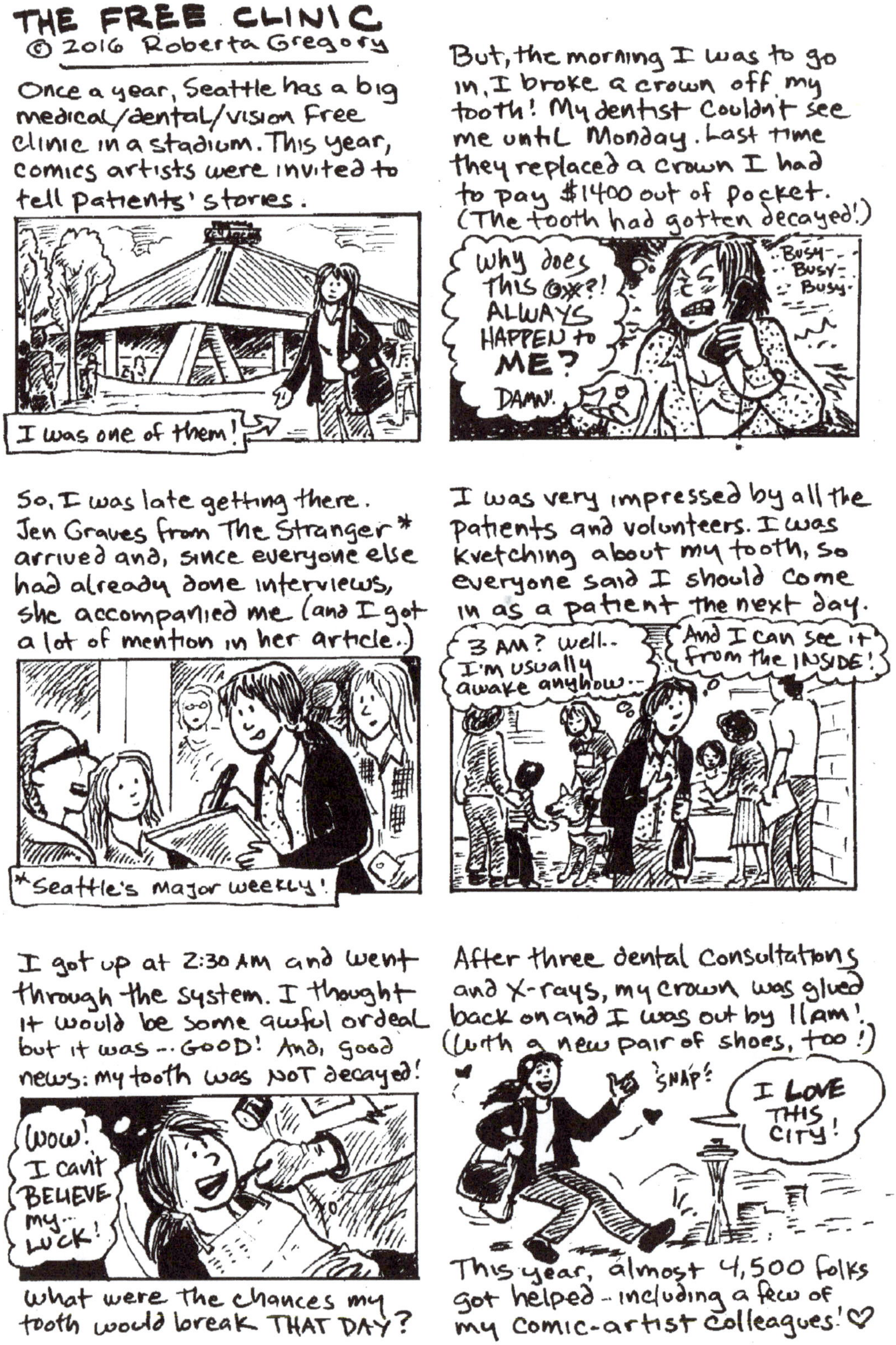
THE FREE CLINIC
© 2016 Roberta Gregory
Once a year, Seattle has a big medical/dental/vision free clinic in a stadium. This year, comics artists were invited to tell patients' stories.
I was one of them!
But, the morning I was to go in, I broke a crown off my tooth! My dentist couldn't see me until Monday. Last time they replaced a crown I had to pay $1400 out of pocket. (The tooth had gotten decayed!)
Why does THIS @※?! ALWAYS HAPPEN to ME?
DAMN!
Busy-Busy-Busy-
So, I was late getting there. Jen Graves from The Stranger* arrived and, since everyone else had already done interviews, she accompanied me (and I got a lot of mention in her article.)
*Seattle's major weekly!
I was very impressed by all the patients and volunteers. I was kvetching about my tooth, so everyone said I should come in as a patient the next day.
3 AM? Well.. I'm usually awake anyhow..
And I can see it from the INSIDE!
I got up at 2:30 AM and went through the system. I thought it would be some awful ordeal but it was -- GOOD! And, good news: my tooth was NOT decayed!
WOW! I can't BELIEVE my.. LUCK!
What were the chances my tooth would break THAT DAY?
After three dental consultations and X-rays, my crown was glued back on and I was out by 11 AM! (With a new pair of shoes, too!)
SNAP!
I LOVE THIS CITY!
This year, almost 4,500 folks got helped - including a few of my comic-artist colleagues! ♡

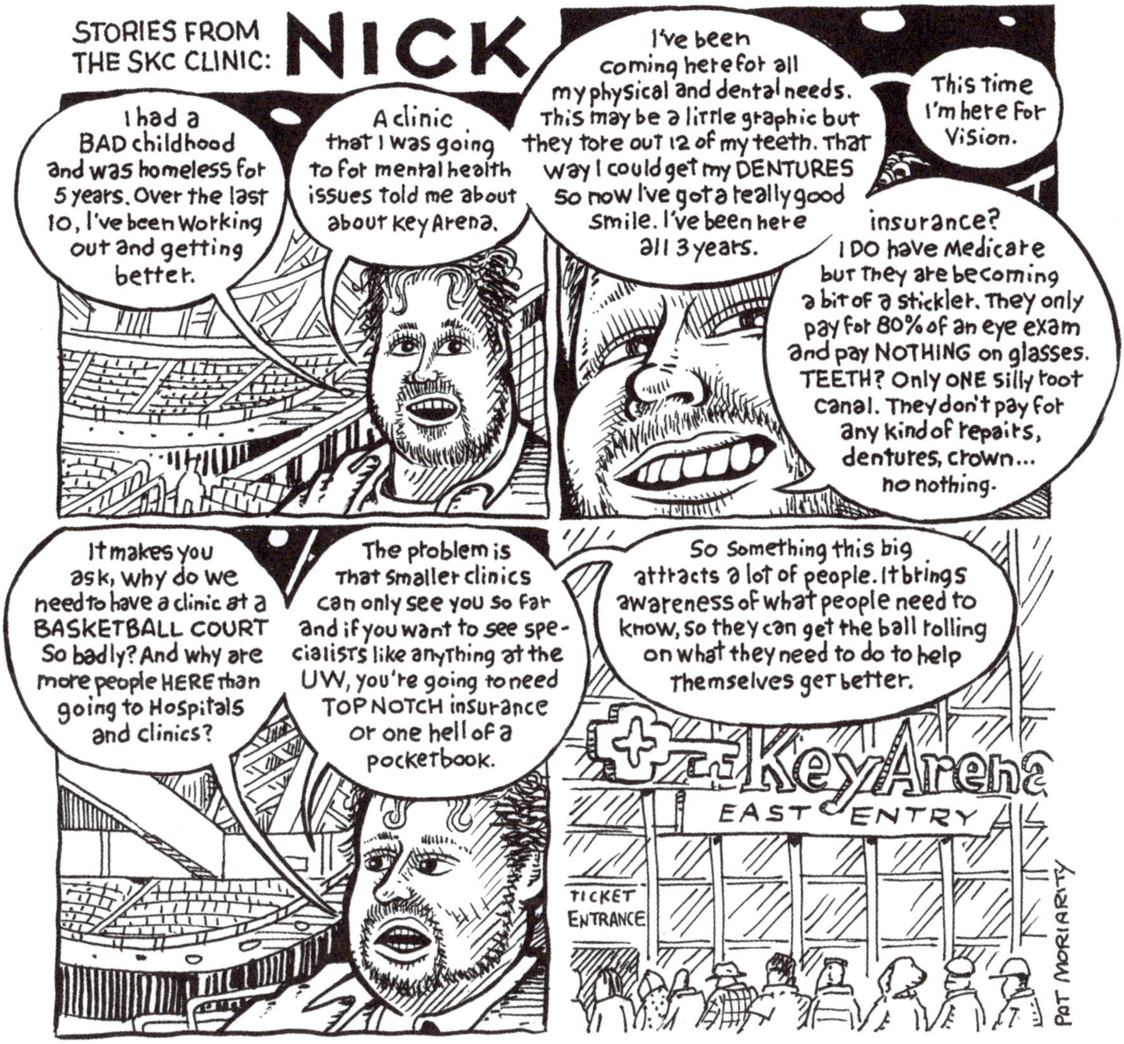

STORIES FROM THE SKC CLINIC: NICK
I had a BAD childhood and was homeless for 5 years. Over the last 10, I've been working out and getting better.
A clinic that I was going to for mental health issues told me about about Key Arena.
I've been coming here for all my physical and dental needs. This may be a little graphic but they tore out 12 of my teeth. That way I could get my DENTURES so now I've got a really good smile. I've been here all 3 years.
This time I'm here for Vision.
insurance? I DO have Medicare but they are becoming a bit of a stickler. They only pay for 80% of an eye exam and pay NOTHING on glasses. TEETH? Only ONE silly root canal. They don't pay for any kind of repairs, dentures, crown... no nothing.
It makes you ask, why do we need to have a clinic at a BASKETBALL COURT so badly? And why are more people HERE than going to Hospitals and clinics?
The problem is that smaller clinics can only see you so far and if you want to see specialists like anything at the UW, you're going to need TOP NOTCH insurance or one hell of a pocketbook.
So something this big attracts a lot of people. It brings awareness of what people need to know, so they can get the ball rolling on what they need to do to help themselves get better.
KeyArena
EAST ENTRY
TICKET ENTRANCE
PAT MORIARITY

The Lottery

Kelly Froh

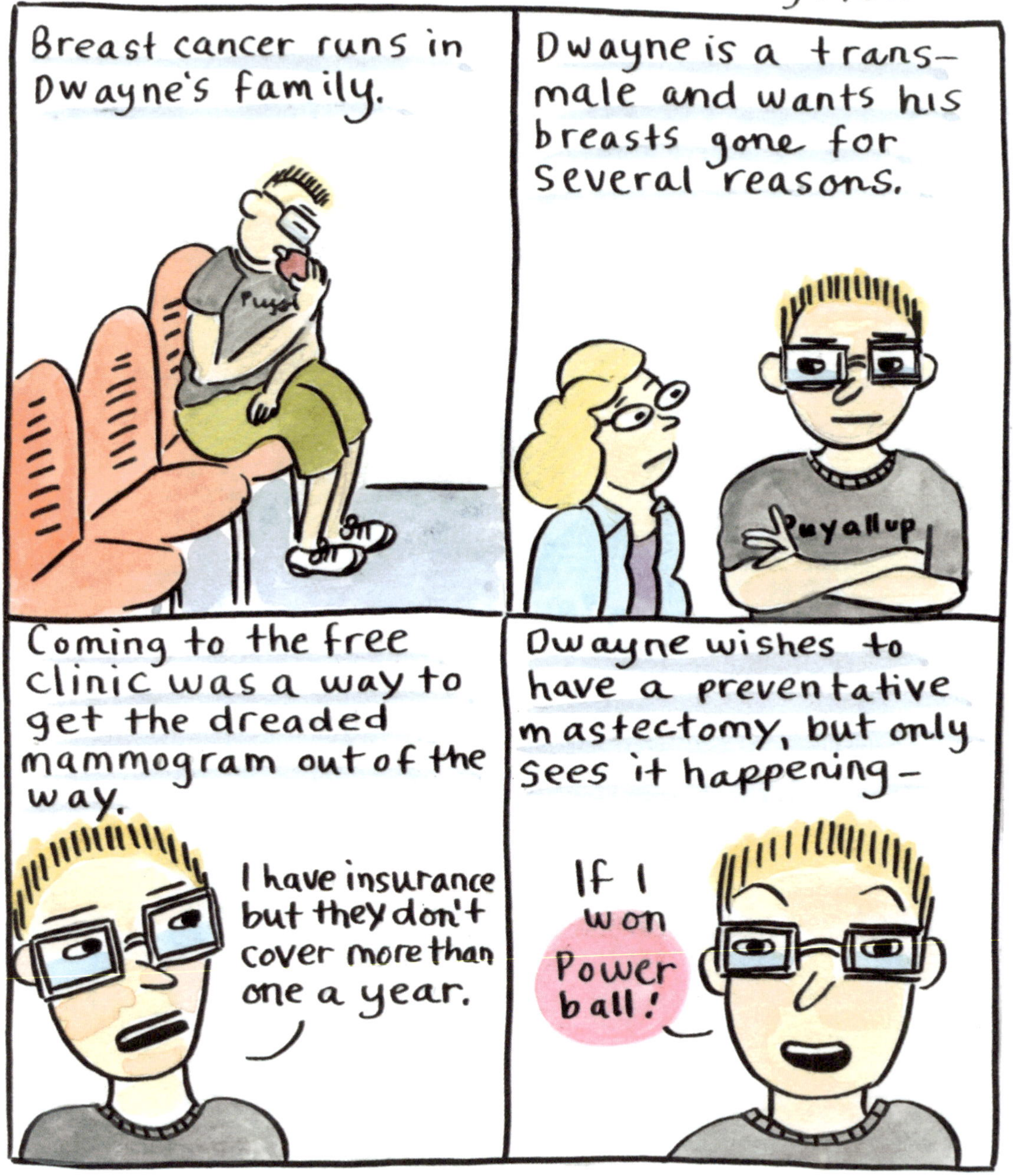
Breast cancer runs in Dwayne's family.
Dwayne is a trans-male and wants his breasts gone for several reasons.
Puyallup
Coming to the free clinic was a way to get the dreaded mammogram out of the way.
I have insurance but they don't cover more than one a year.
Dwayne wishes to have a preventative mastectomy, but only sees it happening–
If I won Powerball!

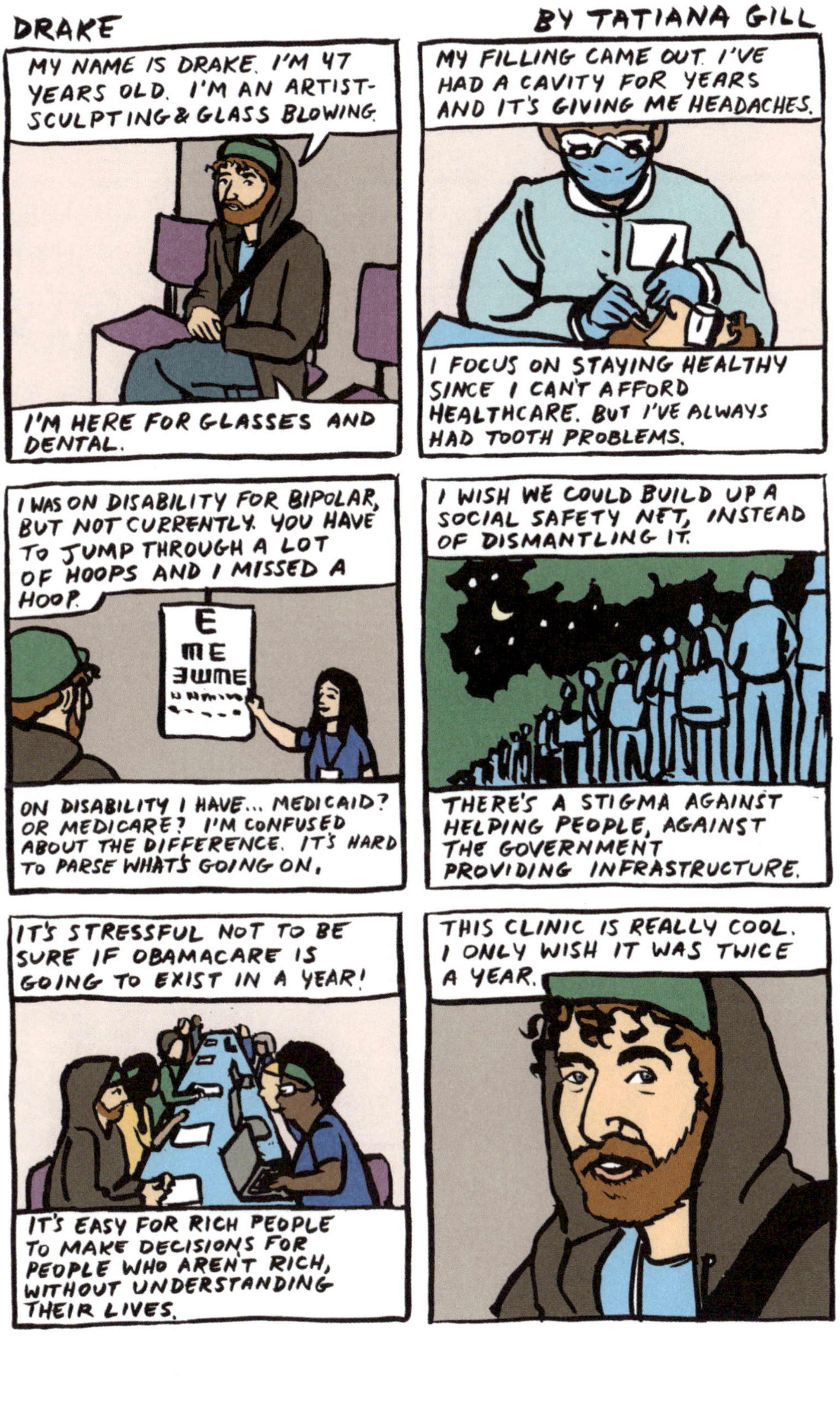
DRAKE
BY TATIANA GILL
MY NAME IS DRAKE. I'M 47 YEARS OLD. I'M AN ARTIST- SCULPTING & GLASS BLOWING.
I'M HERE FOR GLASSES AND DENTAL.
MY FILLING CAME OUT. I'VE HAD A CAVITY FOR YEARS AND IT'S GIVING ME HEADACHES.
I FOCUS ON STAYING HEALTHY SINCE I CAN'T AFFORD HEALTHCARE. BUT I'VE ALWAYS HAD TOOTH PROBLEMS.
I WAS ON DISABILITY FOR BIPOLAR, BUT NOT CURRENTLY. YOU HAVE TO JUMP THROUGH A LOT OF HOOPS AND I MISSED A HOOP.
E
ME
ƎWME
ON DISABILITY I HAVE... MEDICAID? OR MEDICARE? I'M CONFUSED ABOUT THE DIFFERENCE. IT'S HARD TO PARSE WHAT'S GOING ON.
I WISH WE COULD BUILD UP A SOCIAL SAFETY NET, INSTEAD OF DISMANTLING IT.
THERE'S A STIGMA AGAINST HELPING PEOPLE, AGAINST THE GOVERNMENT PROVIDING INFRASTRUCTURE.
IT'S STRESSFUL NOT TO BE SURE IF OBAMACARE IS GOING TO EXIST IN A YEAR!
IT'S EASY FOR RICH PEOPLE TO MAKE DECISIONS FOR PEOPLE WHO AREN'T RICH, WITHOUT UNDERSTANDING THEIR LIVES.
THIS CLINIC IS REALLY COOL. I ONLY WISH IT WAS TWICE A YEAR.

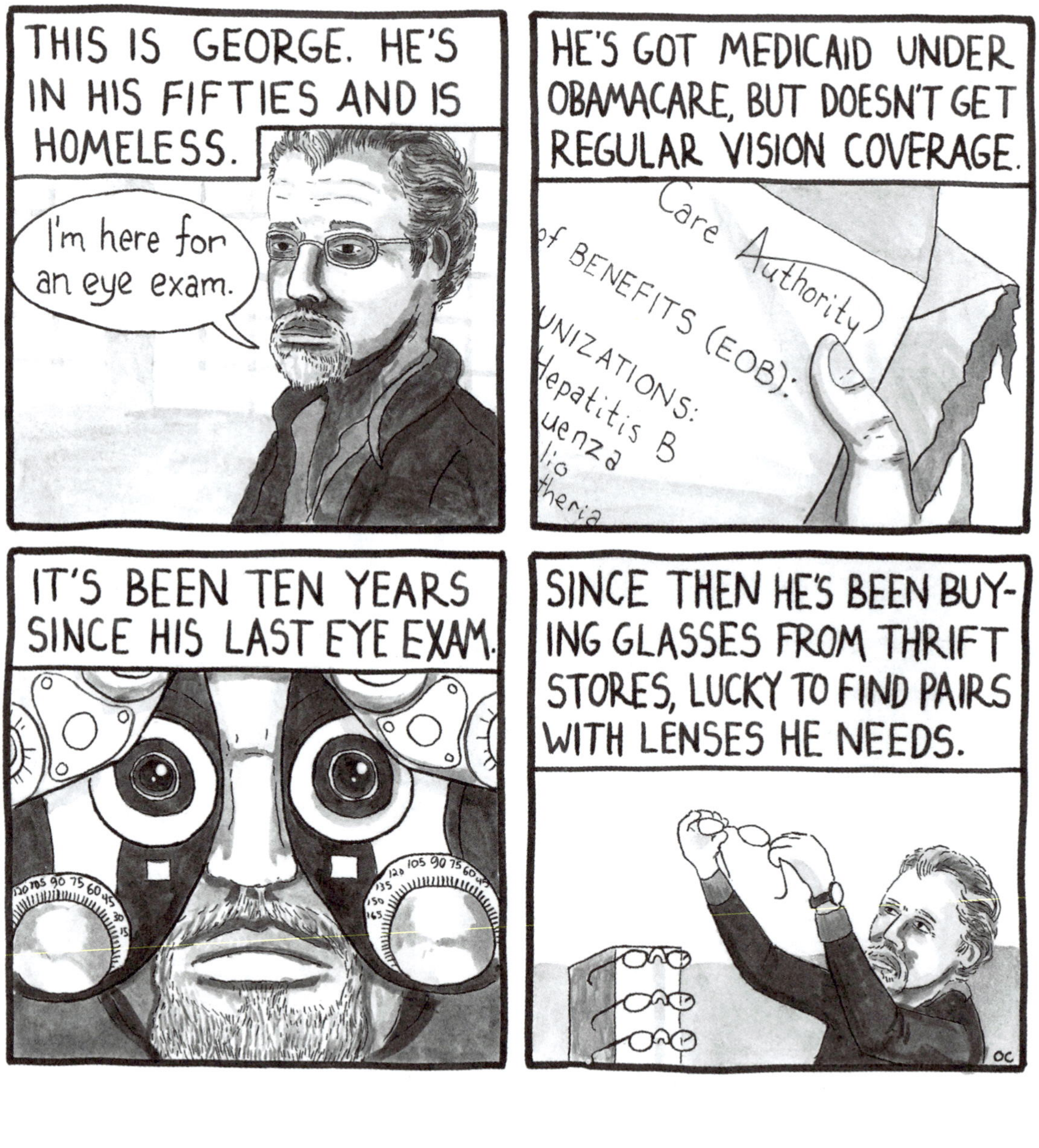

THIS IS GEORGE. HE'S IN HIS FIFTIES AND IS HOMELESS.
I'm here for an eye exam.
HE'S GOT MEDICAID UNDER OBAMACARE, BUT DOESN'T GET REGULAR VISION COVERAGE.
Care Authority
of BENEFITS (EOB):
UNIZATIONS:
Hepatitis B
uenza
lio
theria
IT'S BEEN TEN YEARS SINCE HIS LAST EYE EXAM.
SINCE THEN HE'S BEEN BUYING GLASSES FROM THRIFT STORES, LUCKY TO FIND PAIRS WITH LENSES HE NEEDS.

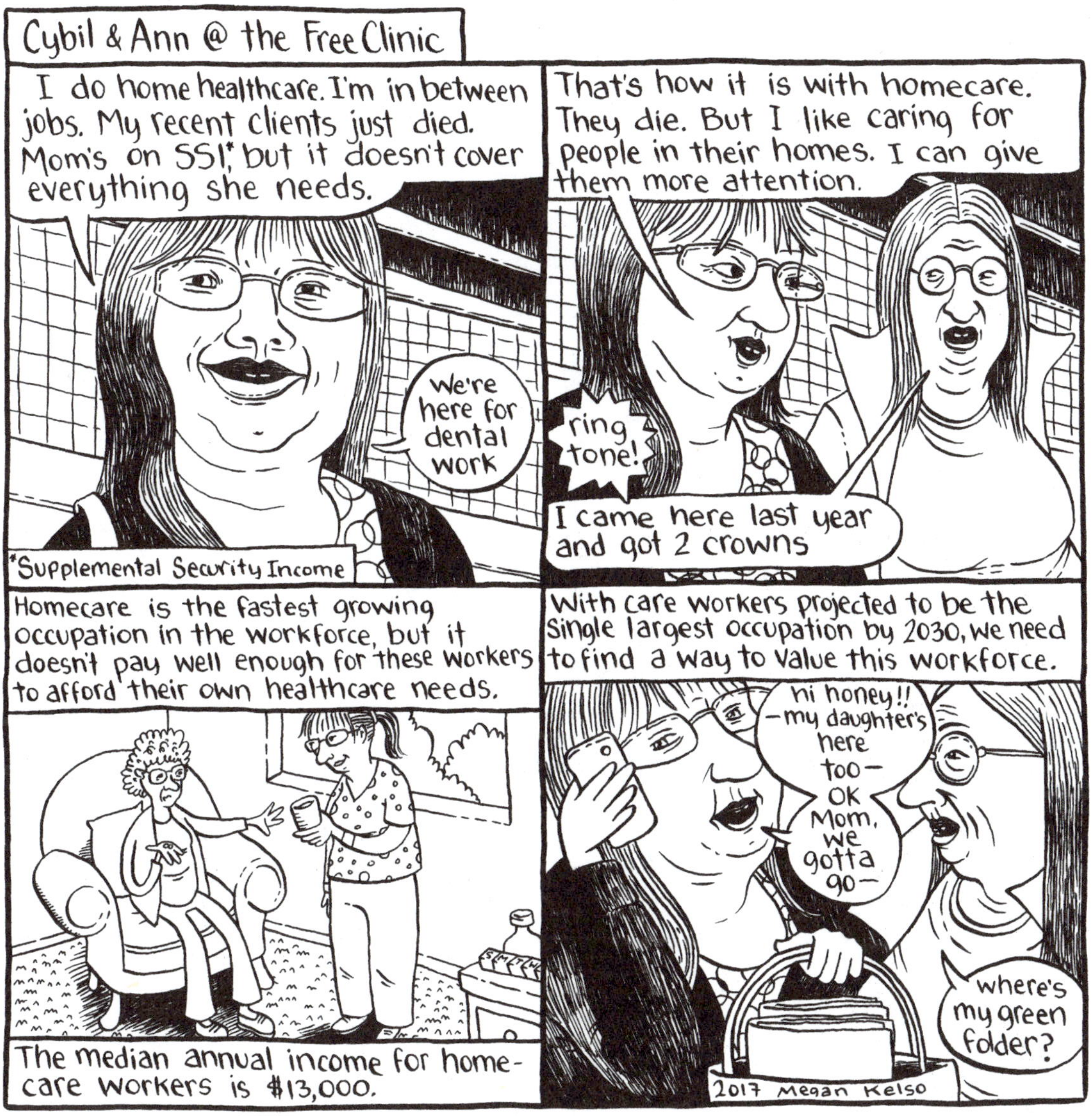

Cybil & Ann @ the Free Clinic
I do home healthcare. I'm in between jobs. My recent clients just died. Mom's on SSI,* but it doesn't cover everything she needs.
We're here for dental work
*Supplemental Security Income
That's how it is with homecare. They die. But I like caring for people in their homes. I can give them more attention.
ring tone!
I came here last year and got 2 crowns
Homecare is the fastest growing occupation in the workforce, but it doesn't pay well enough for these workers to afford their own healthcare needs.
The median annual income for home-care workers is $13,000.
With care workers projected to be the single largest occupation by 2030, we need to find a way to value this workforce.
hi honey!! —my daughter's here too—
OK Mom, we gotta go—
where's my green folder?
2017 Megan Kelso

TAYLOR AND JOSH

BOTH TAYLOR AND JOSH WORK BUT THEIR COMPANY PAYS AN ANNUAL FINE RATHER THAN PROVIDE EMPLOYEES WITH ADEQUATE HEALTH INSURANCE. THEY MAKE TOO MUCH TO QUALIFY FOR MEDICAID BUT CAN ONLY AFFORD TO BUY ONE PLAN THROUGH THE EXCHANGE. BECAUSE JOSH NEEDS A MONTHLY PRESCRIPTION, HE'S THE ONE WITH INSURANCE. NEITHER HAVE DENTAL COVERAGE.

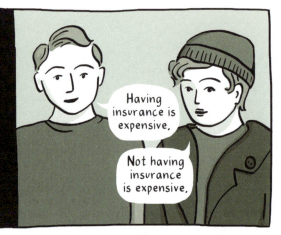

Having insurance is expensive.

Not having insurance is expensive.

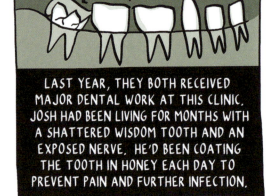

LAST YEAR, THEY BOTH RECEIVED MAJOR DENTAL WORK AT THIS CLINIC. JOSH HAD BEEN LIVING FOR MONTHS WITH A SHATTERED WISDOM TOOTH AND AN EXPOSED NERVE. HE'D BEEN COATING THE TOOTH IN HONEY EACH DAY TO PREVENT PAIN AND FURTHER INFECTION.

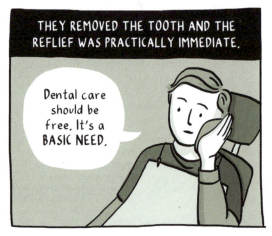

THEY REMOVED THE TOOTH AND THE REFLIEF WAS PRACTICALLY IMMEDIATE.

Dental care should be free. It's a BASIC NEED.

TO PREVENT A POSSIBLE EXTRACTION LAST YEAR, TAYLOR HAD A TOOTH FILED DOWN AND WAS GIVEN PRESCRIPTION TOOTHPASTE.

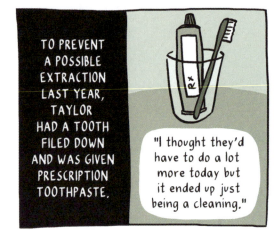

"I thought they'd have to do a lot more today but it ended up just being a cleaning."

TAYLOR USED HER EXTRA TIME TO HAVE A PHYSICAL EXAM AND BLOOD WORK DONE. NEXT, THEY WERE GOING TO TALK WITH A VOLUNTEER ABOUT INSURANCE OPTIONS.

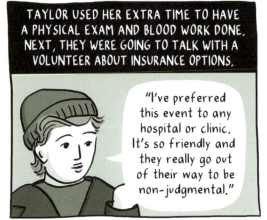

"I've preferred this event to any hospital or clinic. It's so friendly and they really go out of their way to be non-judgmental."

A. CAMBER

DAVE

BY TATIANA GILL

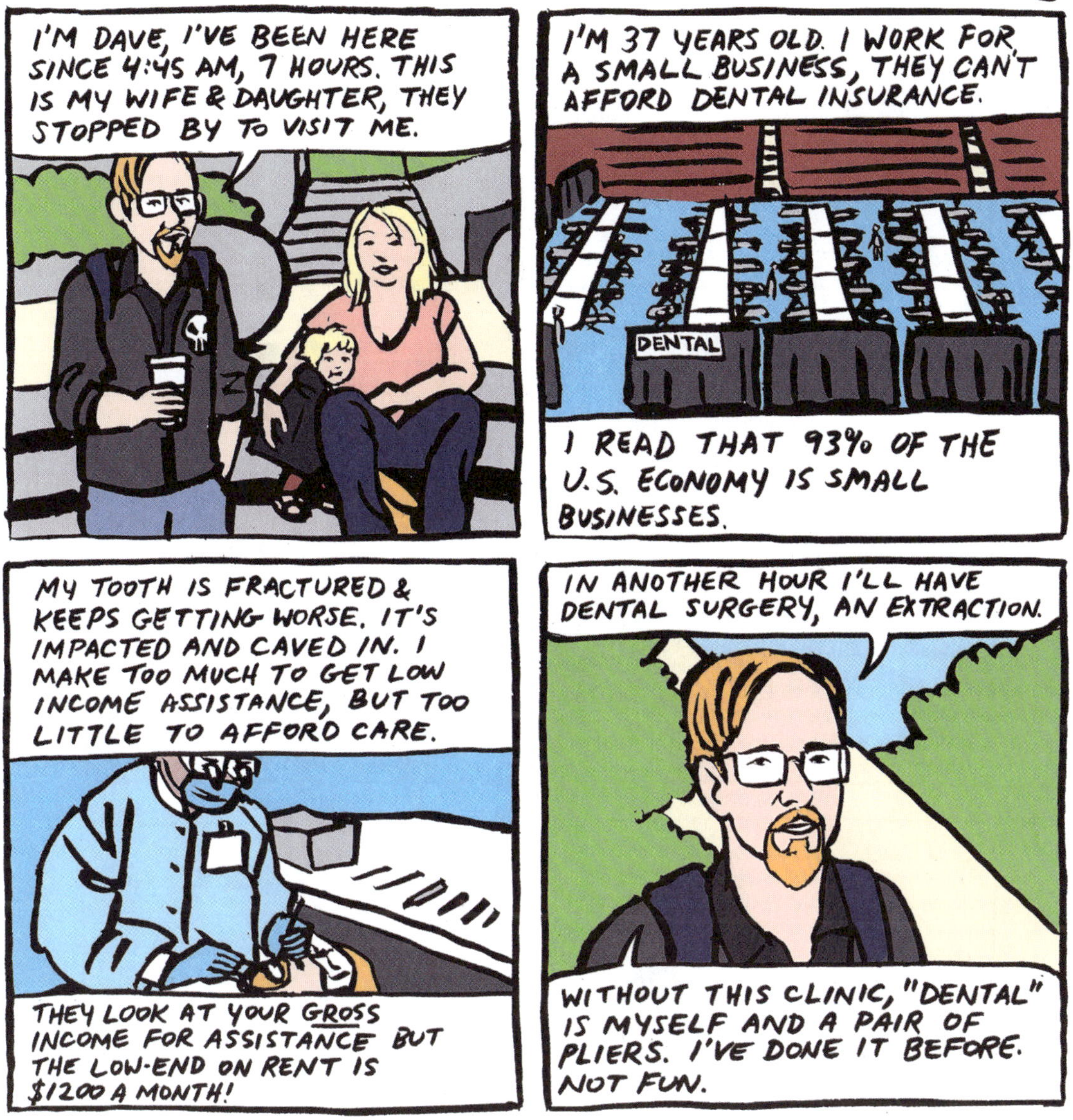
I'M DAVE, I'VE BEEN HERE SINCE 4:45 AM, 7 HOURS. THIS IS MY WIFE & DAUGHTER, THEY STOPPED BY TO VISIT ME.
I'M 37 YEARS OLD. I WORK FOR A SMALL BUSINESS, THEY CAN'T AFFORD DENTAL INSURANCE.
DENTAL
I READ THAT 93% OF THE U.S. ECONOMY IS SMALL BUSINESSES.
MY TOOTH IS FRACTURED & KEEPS GETTING WORSE. IT'S IMPACTED AND CAVED IN. I MAKE TOO MUCH TO GET LOW INCOME ASSISTANCE, BUT TOO LITTLE TO AFFORD CARE.
THEY LOOK AT YOUR GROSS INCOME FOR ASSISTANCE BUT THE LOW-END ON RENT IS $1200 A MONTH!
IN ANOTHER HOUR I'LL HAVE DENTAL SURGERY, AN EXTRACTION.
WITHOUT THIS CLINIC, "DENTAL" IS MYSELF AND A PAIR OF PLIERS. I'VE DONE IT BEFORE. NOT FUN.

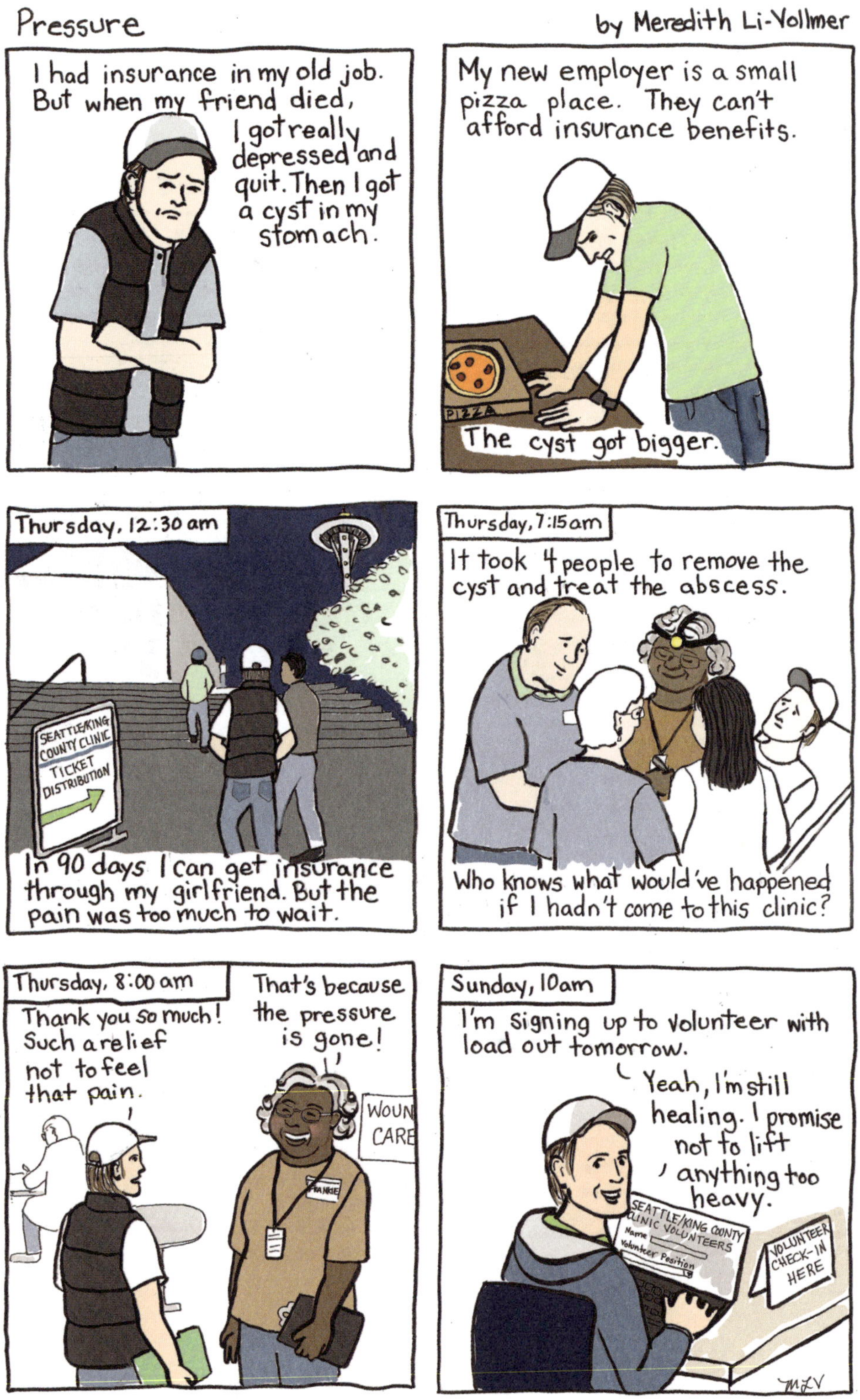
Pressure
by Meredith Li-Vollmer
I had insurance in my old job. But when my friend died, I got really depressed and quit. Then I got a cyst in my stomach.
My new employer is a small pizza place. They can't afford insurance benefits.
PIZZA
The cyst got bigger.
Thursday, 12:30 am
SEATTLE/KING COUNTY CLINIC
TICKET DISTRIBUTION
In 90 days I can get insurance through my girlfriend. But the pain was too much to wait.
Thursday, 7:15 am
It took 4 people to remove the cyst and treat the abscess.
Who knows what would've happened if I hadn't come to this clinic?
Thursday, 8:00 am
Thank you so much! Such a relief not to feel that pain.
That's because the pressure is gone!
FRANKIE
Sunday, 10am
I'm signing up to volunteer with load out tomorrow.
Yeah, I'm still healing. I promise not to lift anything too heavy.
SEATTLE/KING COUNTY CLINIC VOLUNTEERS
Name
Volunteer Position
VOLUNTEER CHECK-IN HERE
MLV

Not Optimistic

by Rachel Scheer

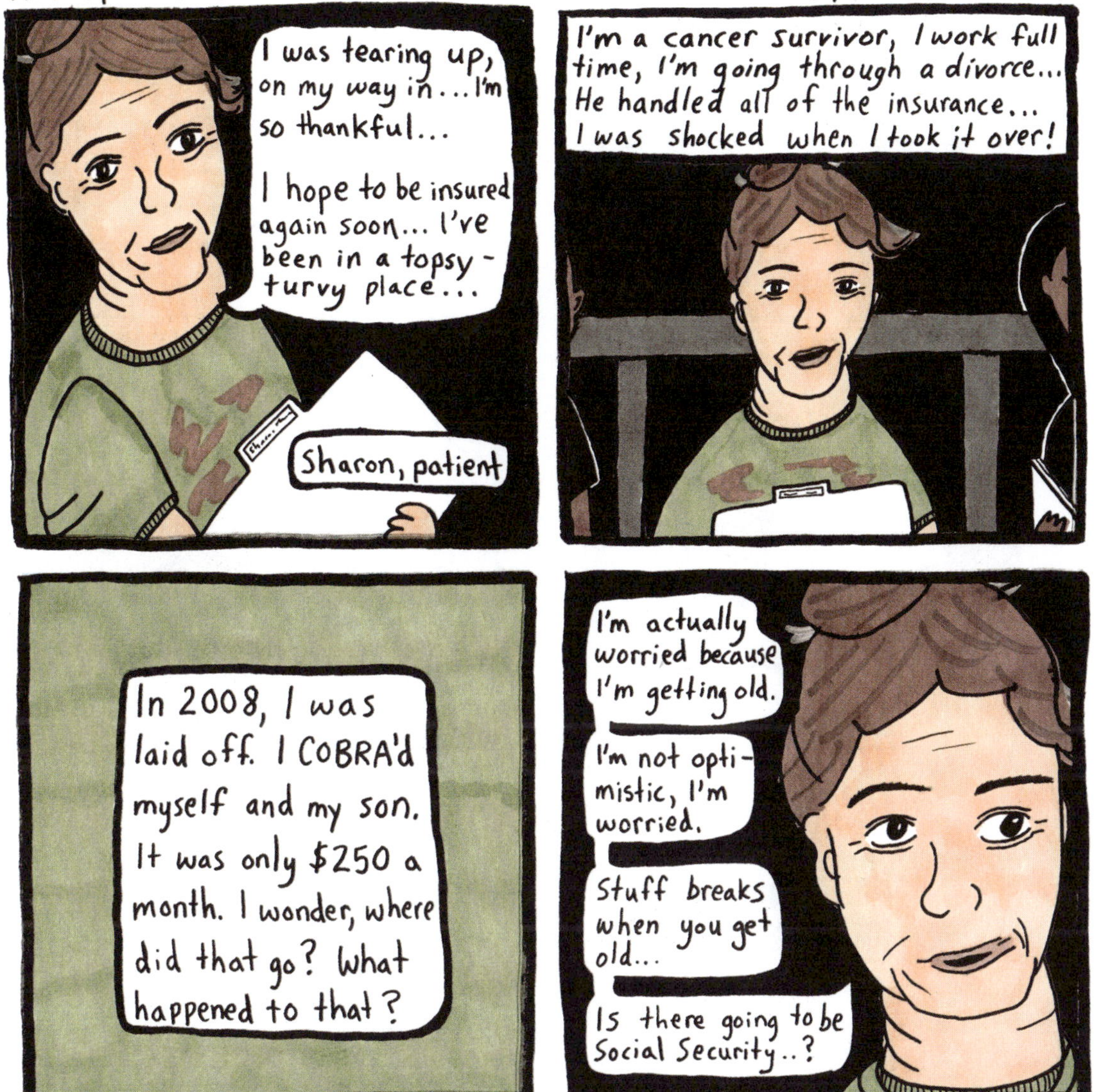
I was tearing up, on my way in... I'm so thankful...
I hope to be insured again soon... I've been in a topsy-turvy place...
Sharon, patient
I'm a cancer survivor, I work full time, I'm going through a divorce... He handled all of the insurance... I was shocked when I took it over!
In 2008, I was laid off. I COBRA'd myself and my son. It was only $250 a month. I wonder, where did that go? What happened to that?
I'm actually worried because I'm getting old.
I'm not optimistic, I'm worried.
Stuff breaks when you get old...
Is there going to be Social Security..?

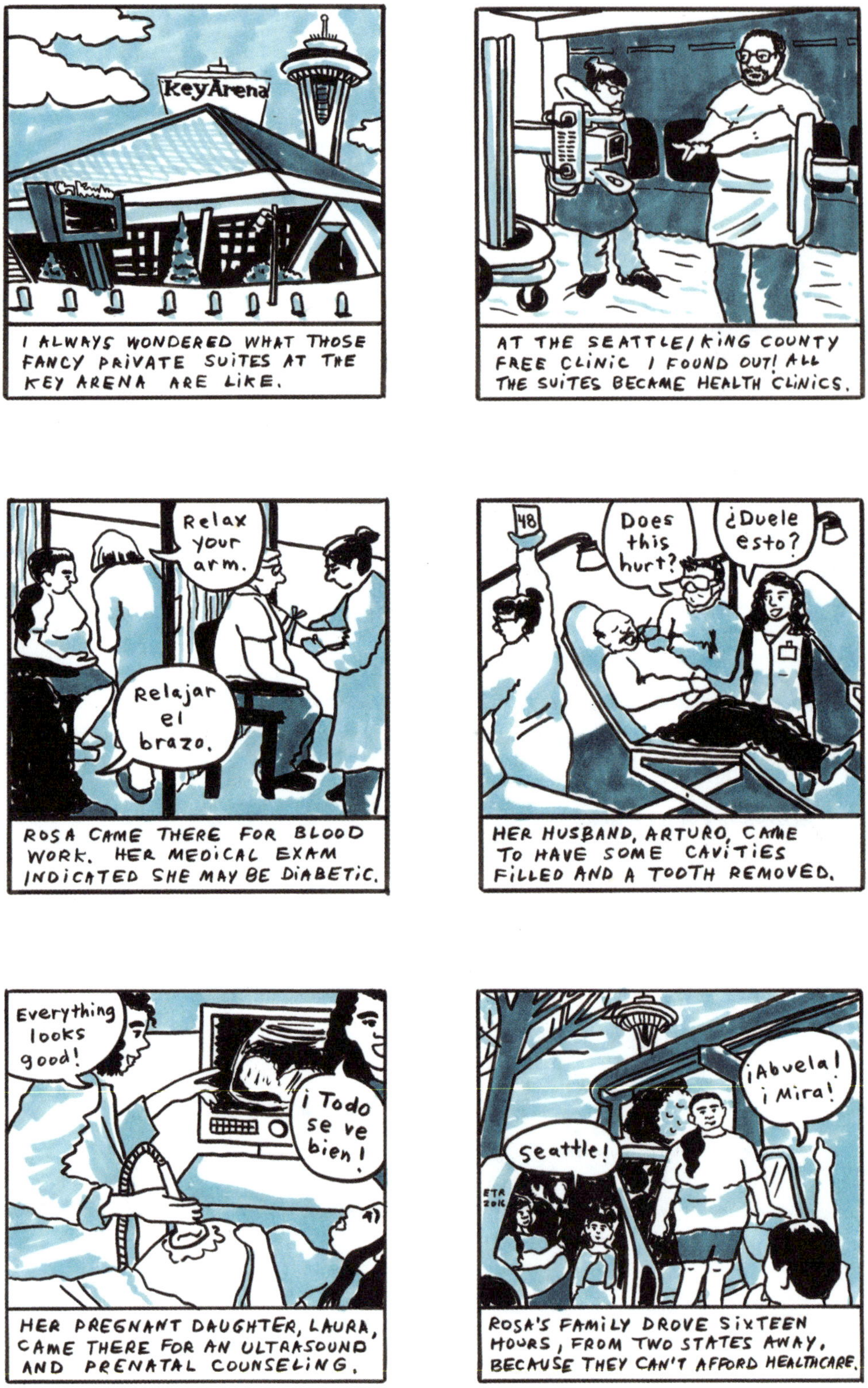

KeyArena
I ALWAYS WONDERED WHAT THOSE FANCY PRIVATE SUITES AT THE KEY ARENA ARE LIKE.
AT THE SEATTLE/KING COUNTY FREE CLINIC I FOUND OUT! ALL THE SUITES BECAME HEALTH CLINICS.
Relax your arm.
Relajar el brazo.
ROSA CAME THERE FOR BLOOD WORK. HER MEDICAL EXAM INDICATED SHE MAY BE DIABETIC.
48
Does this hurt?
¿Duele esto?
HER HUSBAND, ARTURO, CAME TO HAVE SOME CAVITIES FILLED AND A TOOTH REMOVED.
Everything looks good!
¡Todo se ve bien!
HER PREGNANT DAUGHTER, LAURA, CAME THERE FOR AN ULTRASOUND AND PRENATAL COUNSELING.
¡Abuela! ¡Mira!
Seattle!
ETR 2016
ROSA'S FAMILY DROVE SIXTEEN HOURS, FROM TWO STATES AWAY, BECAUSE THEY CAN'T AFFORD HEALTHCARE.

FELIPE

BY TATIANA GILL

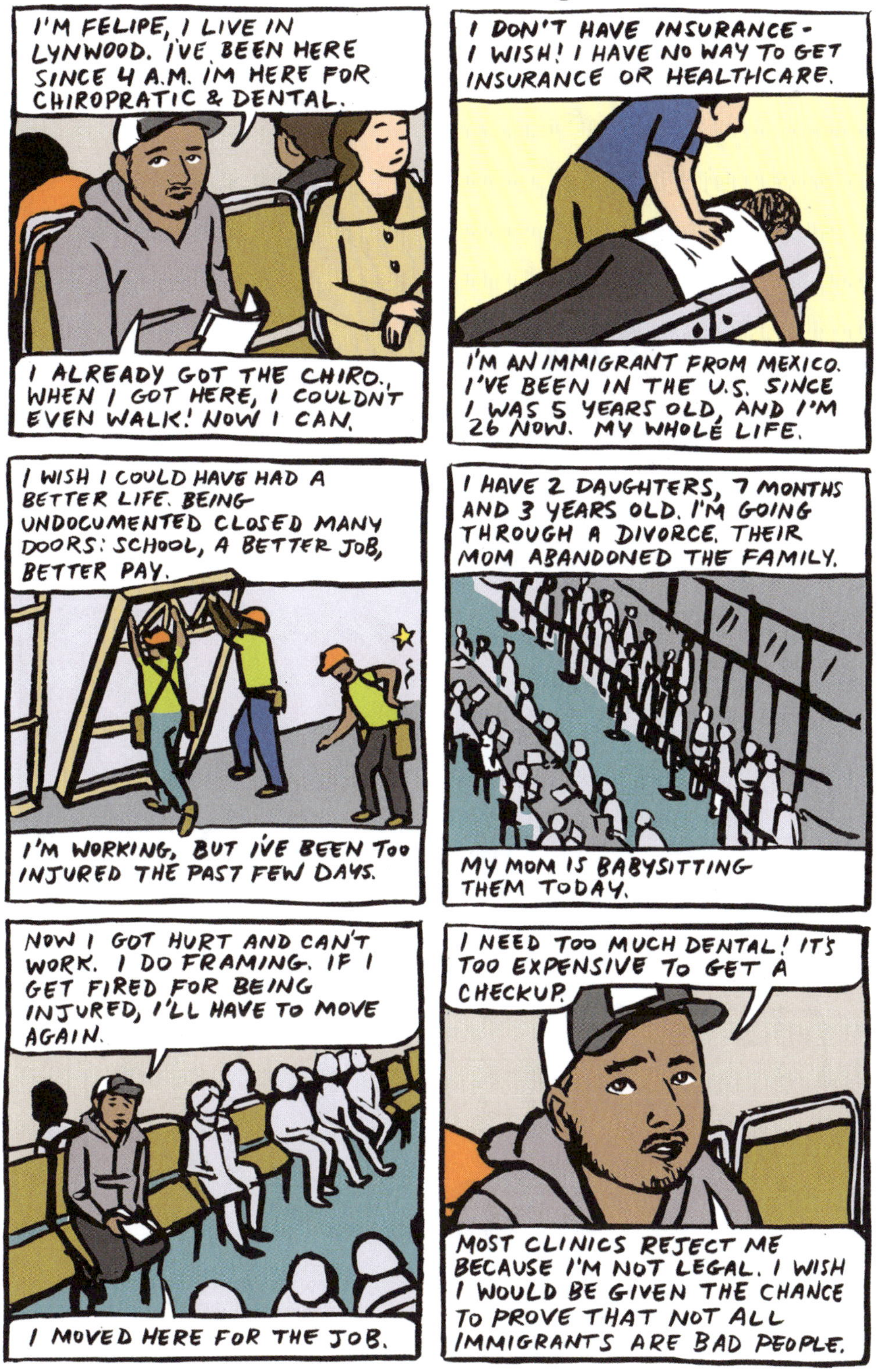

I'M FELIPE, I LIVE IN LYNWOOD. I'VE BEEN HERE SINCE 4 A.M. I'M HERE FOR CHIROPRATIC & DENTAL.
I ALREADY GOT THE CHIRO. WHEN I GOT HERE, I COULDN'T EVEN WALK! NOW I CAN.
I DON'T HAVE INSURANCE - I WISH! I HAVE NO WAY TO GET INSURANCE OR HEALTHCARE.
I'M AN IMMIGRANT FROM MEXICO. I'VE BEEN IN THE U.S. SINCE I WAS 5 YEARS OLD, AND I'M 26 NOW. MY WHOLE LIFE.
I WISH I COULD HAVE HAD A BETTER LIFE. BEING UNDOCUMENTED CLOSED MANY DOORS: SCHOOL, A BETTER JOB, BETTER PAY.
I'M WORKING, BUT I'VE BEEN TOO INJURED THE PAST FEW DAYS.
I HAVE 2 DAUGHTERS, 7 MONTHS AND 3 YEARS OLD. I'M GOING THROUGH A DIVORCE. THEIR MOM ABANDONED THE FAMILY.
MY MOM IS BABYSITTING THEM TODAY.
NOW I GOT HURT AND CAN'T WORK. I DO FRAMING. IF I GET FIRED FOR BEING INJURED, I'LL HAVE TO MOVE AGAIN.
I MOVED HERE FOR THE JOB.
I NEED TOO MUCH DENTAL! IT'S TOO EXPENSIVE TO GET A CHECKUP.
MOST CLINICS REJECT ME BECAUSE I'M NOT LEGAL. I WISH I WOULD BE GIVEN THE CHANCE TO PROVE THAT NOT ALL IMMIGRANTS ARE BAD PEOPLE.

MIXED BLESSING

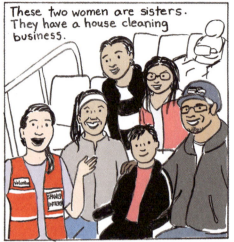

These two women are sisters. They have a house cleaning business.

We get general check-ups at a community health center. We feel blessed and thankful to get our teeth cleaned here.

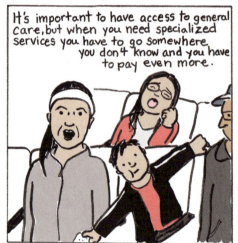

It's important to have access to general care, but when you need specialized services you have to go somewhere you don't know and you have to pay even more.

Look at how her smile lights up because she got dental care here! Immigrants work hard for this country. It's important that we can get health services too.

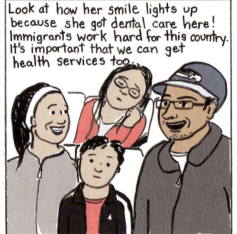

In this country, if you're dying, everything is done for you. They don't want you to die.

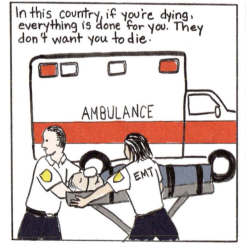

But if you're sick, they charge you. It's very costly.

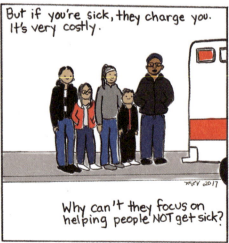

Why can't they focus on helping people NOT get sick?

Imagine

Kelly Froh

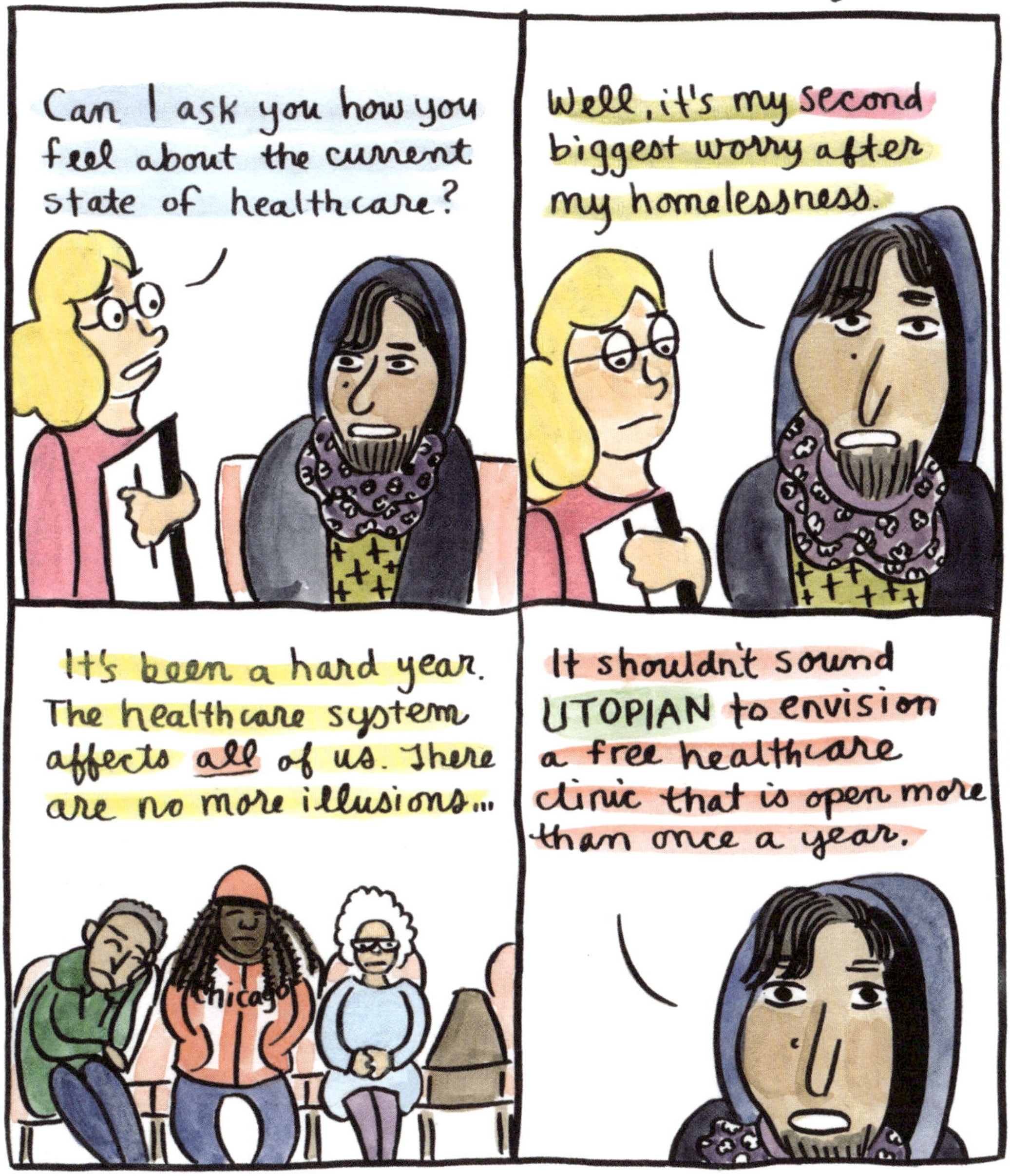
Can I ask you how you feel about the current state of healthcare?
Well, it's my second biggest worry after my homelessness.
It's been a hard year. The healthcare system affects all of us. There are no more illusions...
Chicago
It shouldn't sound UTOPIAN to envision a free healthcare clinic that is open more than once a year.

Ashley, 25 years old

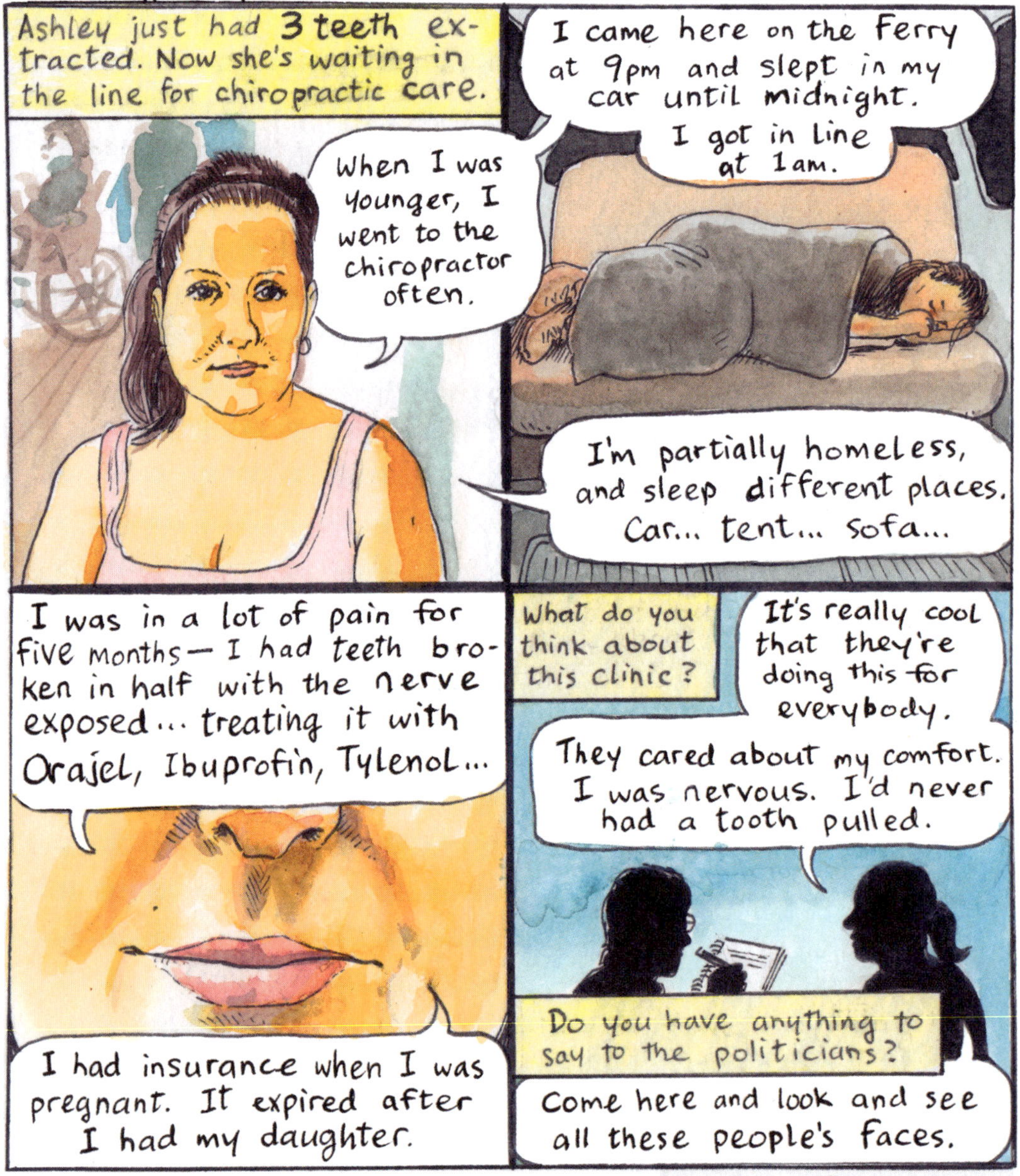

Ashley just had 3 teeth extracted. Now she's waiting in the line for chiropractic care.
When I was younger, I went to the chiropractor often.
I came here on the Ferry at 9pm and slept in my car until midnight.
I got in line at 1am.
I'm partially homeless, and sleep different places. Car... tent... sofa...
I was in a lot of pain for five months— I had teeth broken in half with the nerve exposed... treating it with Orajel, Ibuprofin, Tylenol...
I had insurance when I was pregnant. It expired after I had my daughter.
What do you think about this clinic?
It's really cool that they're doing this for everybody.
They cared about my comfort. I was nervous. I'd never had a tooth pulled.
Do you have anything to say to the politicians?
Come here and look and see all these people's faces.

interview by David Lasky

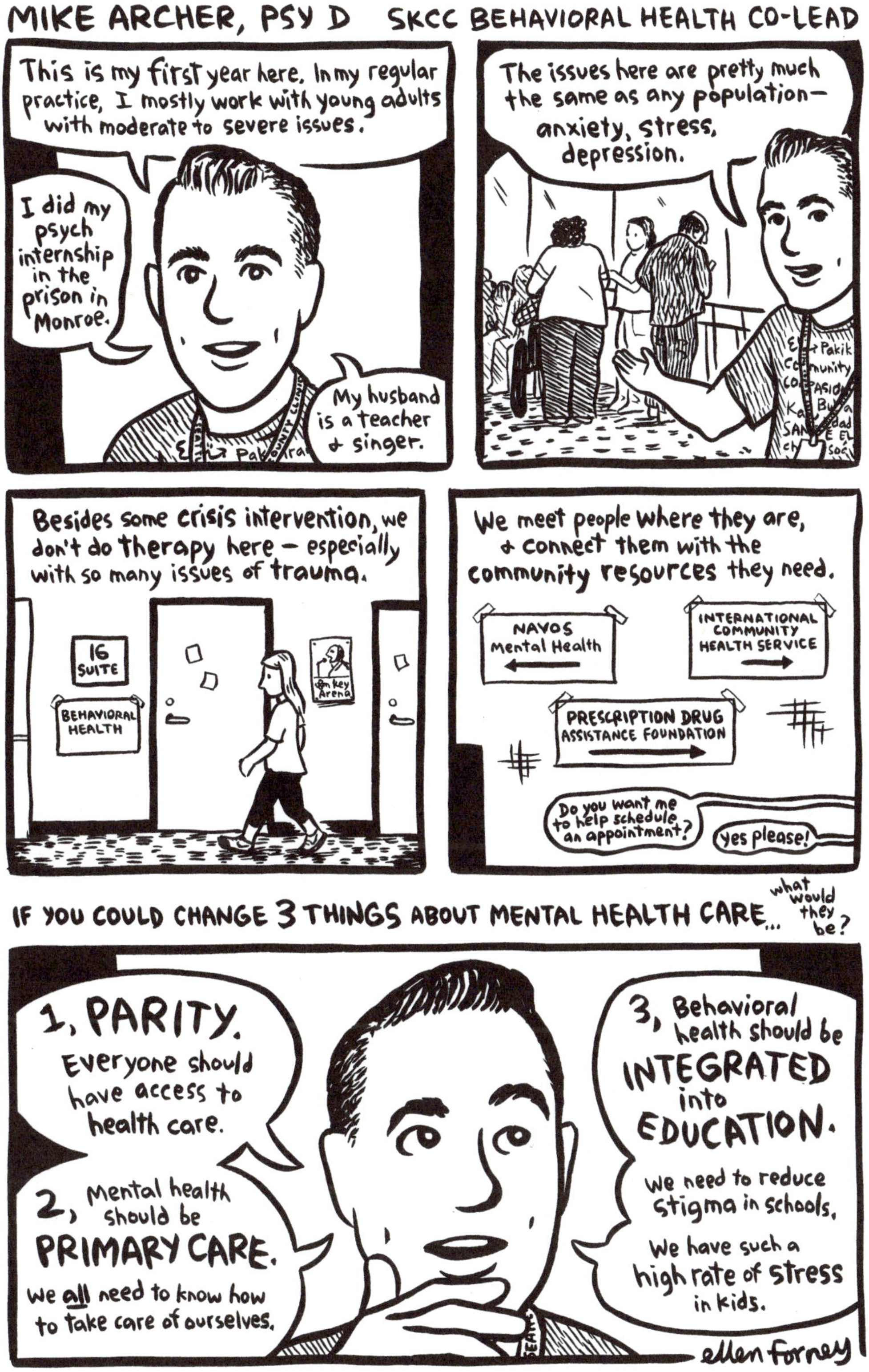
MIKE ARCHER, PSY D SKCC BEHAVIORAL HEALTH CO-LEAD
This is my first year here. In my regular practice, I mostly work with young adults with moderate to severe issues.
I did my psych internship in the prison in Monroe.
My husband is a teacher & singer.
The issues here are pretty much the same as any population— anxiety, stress, depression.
Besides some crisis intervention, we don't do therapy here — especially with so many issues of trauma.
16 SUITE
BEHAVIORAL HEALTH
Key Arena
We meet people where they are, & connect them with the community resources they need.
NAVOS Mental Health
INTERNATIONAL COMMUNITY HEALTH SERVICE
PRESCRIPTION DRUG ASSISTANCE FOUNDATION
Do you want me to help schedule an appointment?
Yes please!
IF YOU COULD CHANGE 3 THINGS ABOUT MENTAL HEALTH CARE... what would they be?
1, PARITY. Everyone should have access to health care.
2, Mental health should be PRIMARY CARE. We all need to know how to take care of ourselves.
3, Behavioral health should be INTEGRATED into EDUCATION. We need to reduce stigma in schools. We have such a high rate of stress in kids.
ellen forney

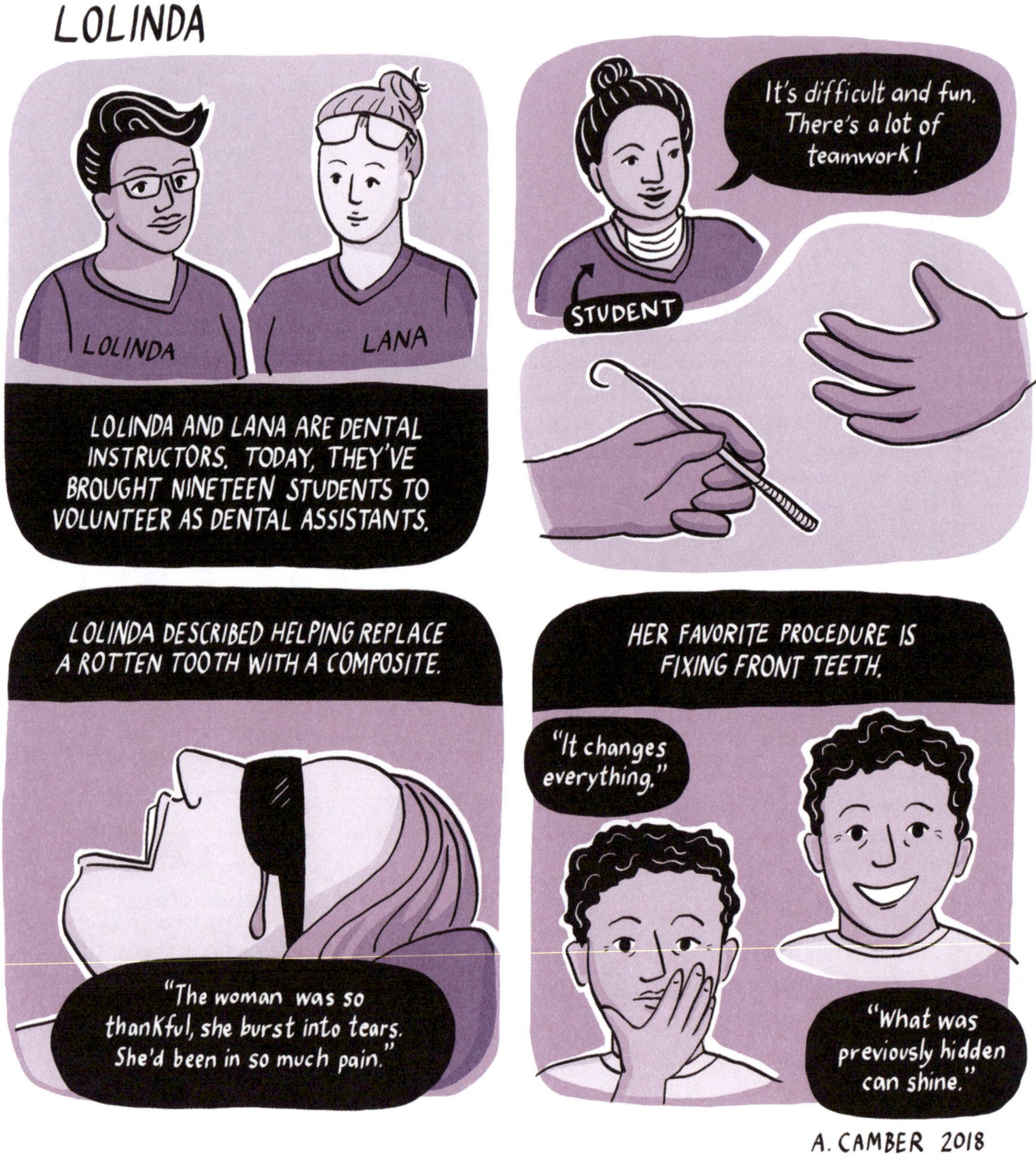
LOLINDA
LOLINDA
LANA
LOLINDA AND LANA ARE DENTAL INSTRUCTORS. TODAY, THEY'VE BROUGHT NINETEEN STUDENTS TO VOLUNTEER AS DENTAL ASSISTANTS.
It's difficult and fun. There's a lot of teamwork!
STUDENT
LOLINDA DESCRIBED HELPING REPLACE A ROTTEN TOOTH WITH A COMPOSITE.
"The woman was so thankful, she burst into tears. She'd been in so much pain."
HER FAVORITE PROCEDURE IS FIXING FRONT TEETH.
"It changes everything."
"What was previously hidden can shine."
A. CAMBER 2018

Health Fair

by Meredith Li-Vollmer

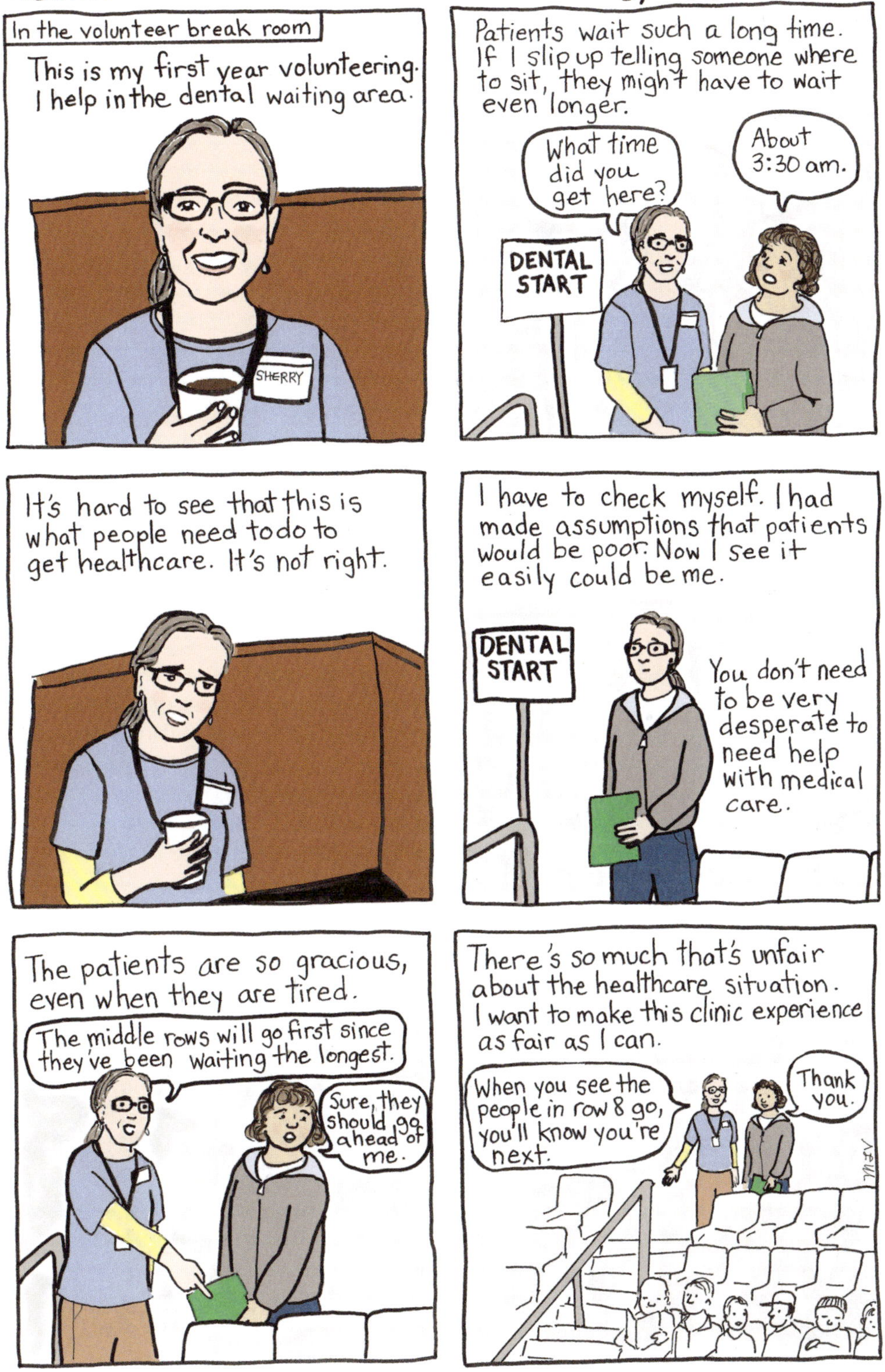
In the volunteer break room
This is my first year volunteering. I help in the dental waiting area.
SHERRY
Patients wait such a long time. If I slip up telling someone where to sit, they might have to wait even longer.
What time did you get here?
About 3:30 am.
DENTAL START
It's hard to see that this is what people need to do to get healthcare. It's not right.
I have to check myself. I had made assumptions that patients would be poor. Now I see it easily could be me.
DENTAL START
You don't need to be very desperate to need help with medical care.
The patients are so gracious, even when they are tired.
The middle rows will go first since they've been waiting the longest.
Sure, they should go ahead of me.
There's so much that's unfair about the healthcare situation. I want to make this clinic experience as fair as I can.
When you see the people in row 8 go, you'll know you're next.
Thank you.

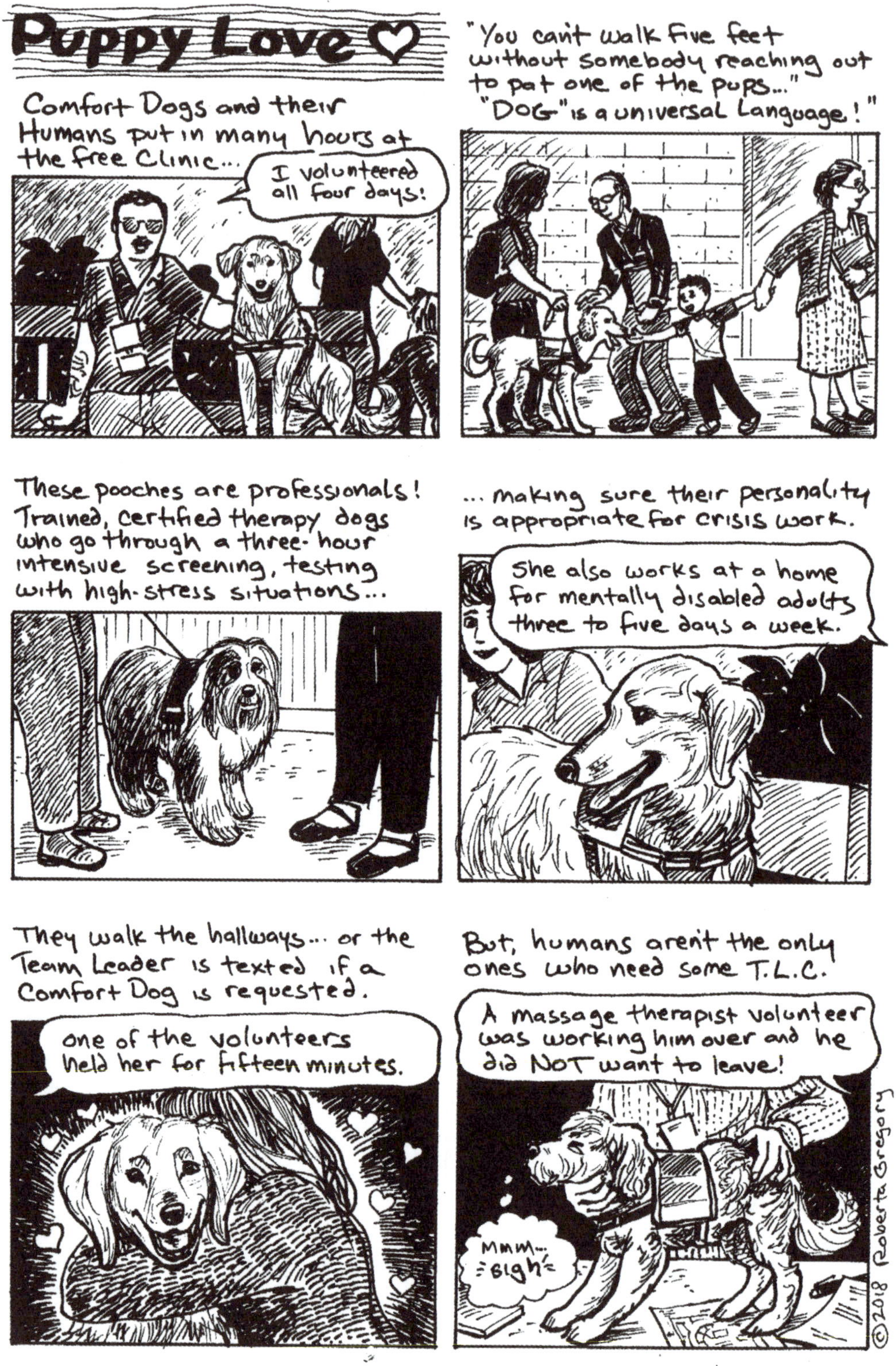
Puppy Love ♡
Comfort Dogs and their Humans put in many hours at the free Clinic...
I volunteered all four days!
"You can't walk five feet without somebody reaching out to pat one of the pups..." "DOG" is a universal Language!"
These pooches are professionals! Trained, certified therapy dogs who go through a three-hour intensive screening, testing with high-stress situations...
...making sure their personality is appropriate for crisis work.
She also works at a home for mentally disabled adults three to five days a week.
They walk the hallways... or the Team Leader is texted if a Comfort Dog is requested.
one of the volunteers held her for fifteen minutes.
But, humans aren't the only ones who need some T.L.C.
A massage therapist volunteer was working him over and he did NOT want to leave!
MMM... SIGH
©2018 Roberta Gregory

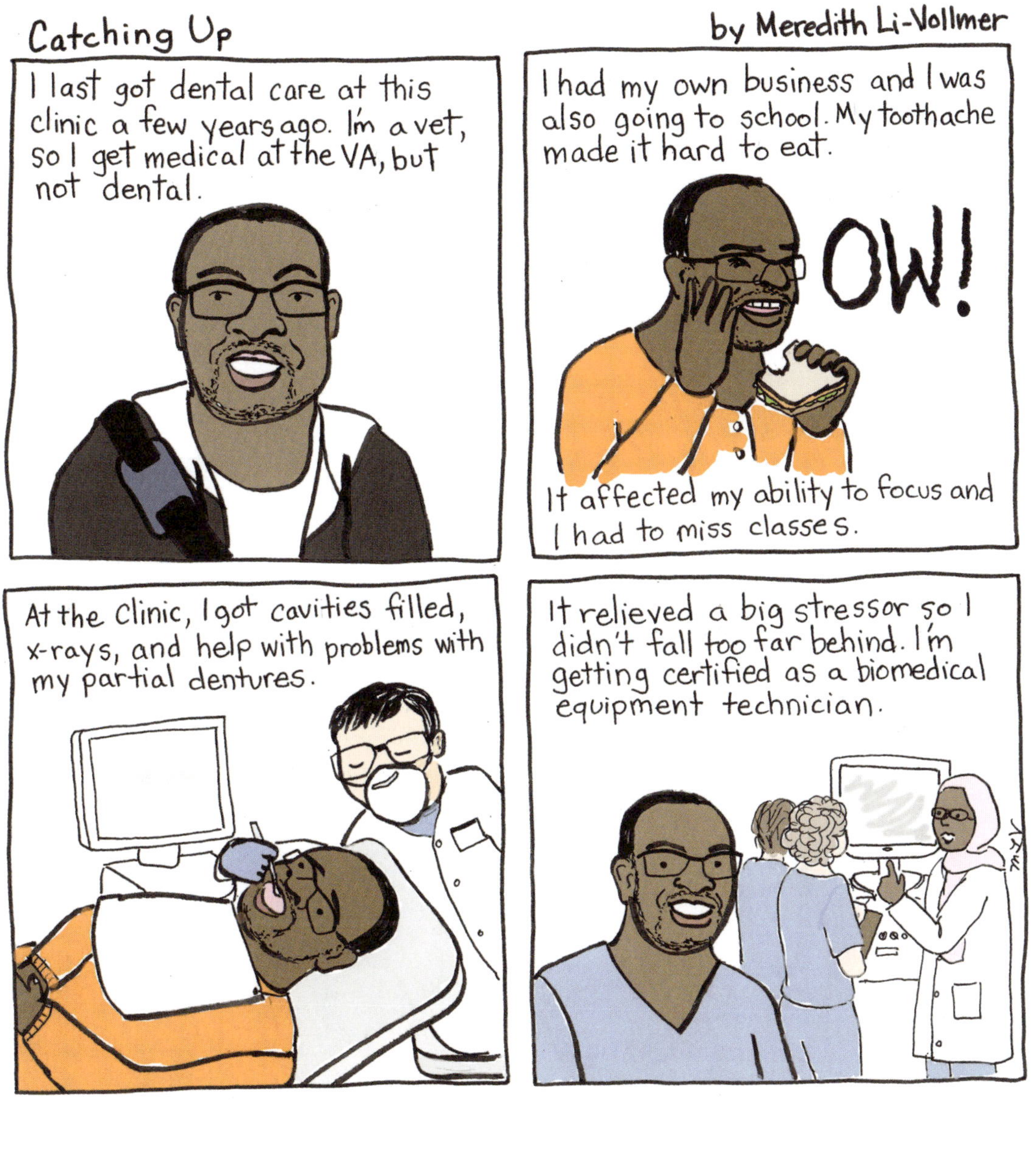
Catching Up
by Meredith Li-Vollmer
I last got dental care at this clinic a few years ago. I'm a vet, so I get medical at the VA, but not dental.
I had my own business and I was also going to school. My toothache made it hard to eat.
OW!
It affected my ability to focus and I had to miss classes.
At the Clinic, I got cavities filled, x-rays, and help with problems with my partial dentures.
It relieved a big stressor so I didn't fall too far behind. I'm getting certified as a biomedical equipment technician.

FOR JANET

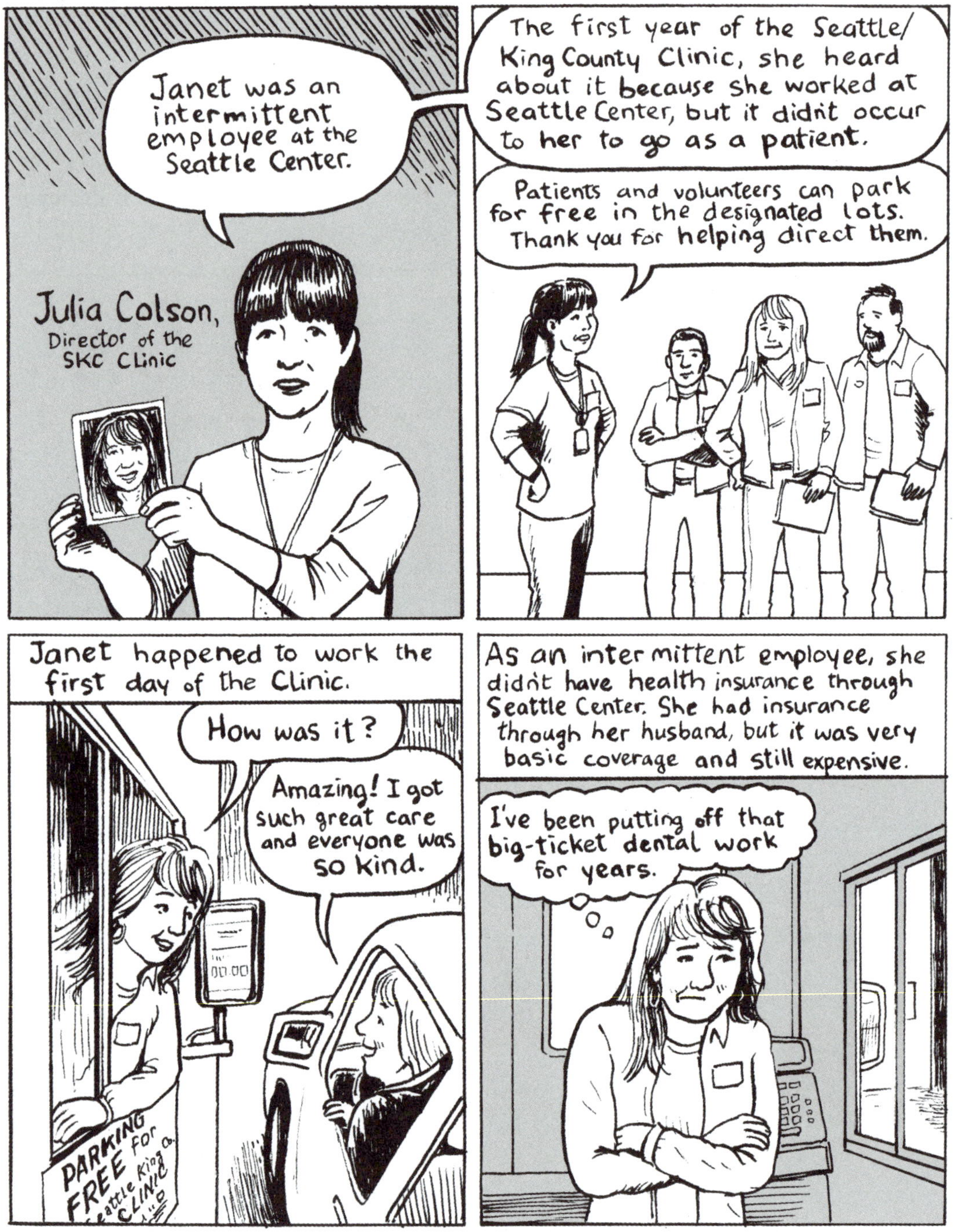
Janet was an intermittent employee at the Seattle Center.
Julia Colson, Director of the SKC Clinic
The first year of the Seattle/King County Clinic, she heard about it because she worked at Seattle Center, but it didn't occur to her to go as a patient.
Patients and volunteers can park for free in the designated lots. Thank you for helping direct them.
Janet happened to work the first day of the Clinic.
How was it?
Amazing! I got such great care and everyone was so kind.
PARKING FREE For Seattle King Co. CLINIC
As an intermittent employee, she didn't have health insurance through Seattle Center. She had insurance through her husband, but it was very basic coverage and still expensive.
I've been putting off that big-ticket dental work for years.

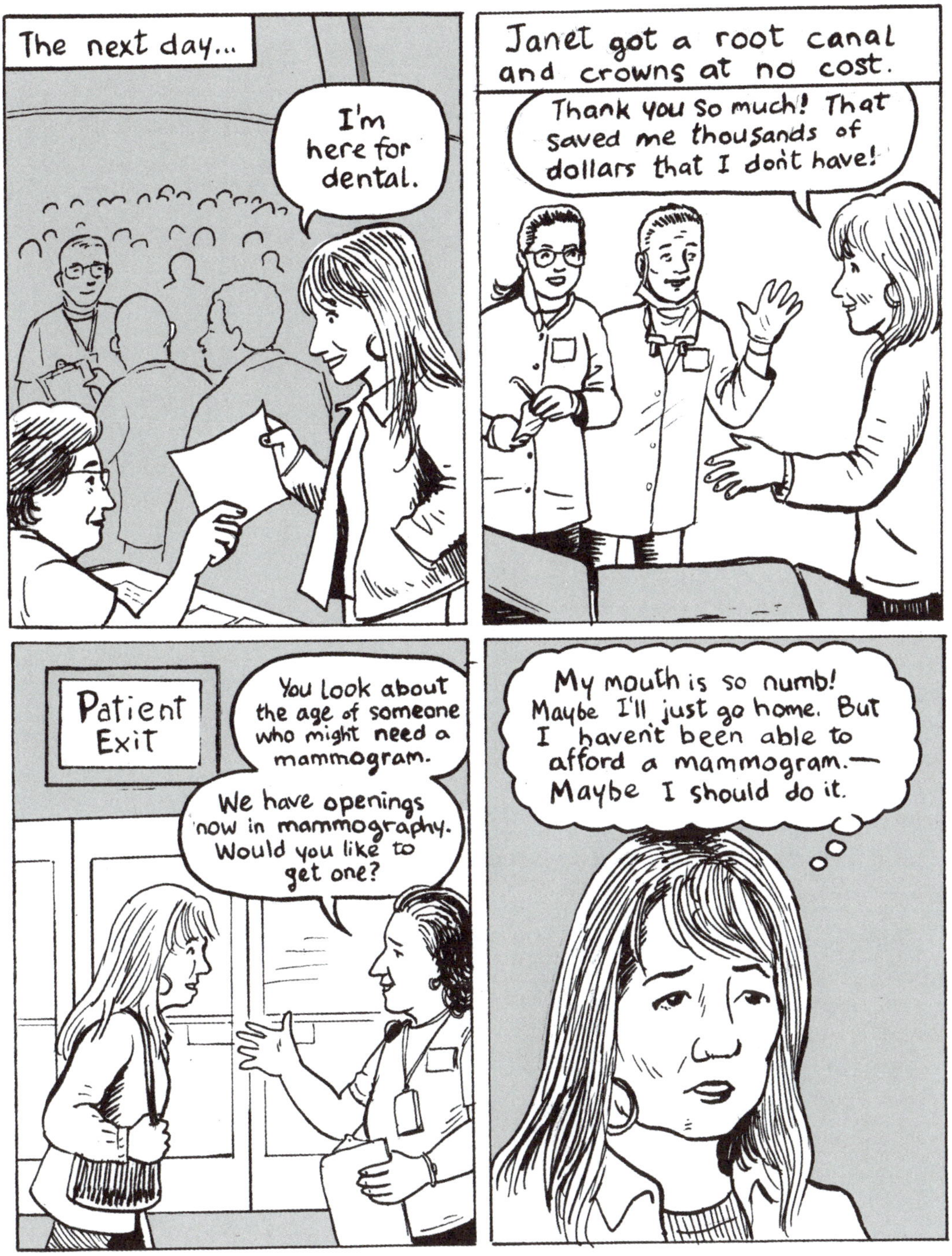
The next day...
I'm here for dental.
Janet got a root canal and crowns at no cost.
Thank you so much! That saved me thousands of dollars that I don't have!
Patient Exit
You look about the age of someone who might need a mammogram.
We have openings now in mammography. Would you like to get one?
My mouth is so numb! Maybe I'll just go home. But I haven't been able to afford a mammogram.— Maybe I should do it.

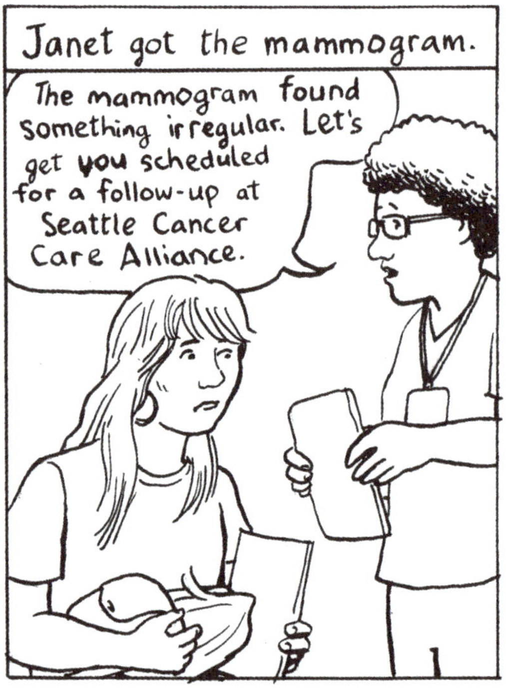
Janet got the mammogram.
The mammogram found something irregular. Let's get you scheduled for a follow-up at Seattle Cancer Care Alliance.

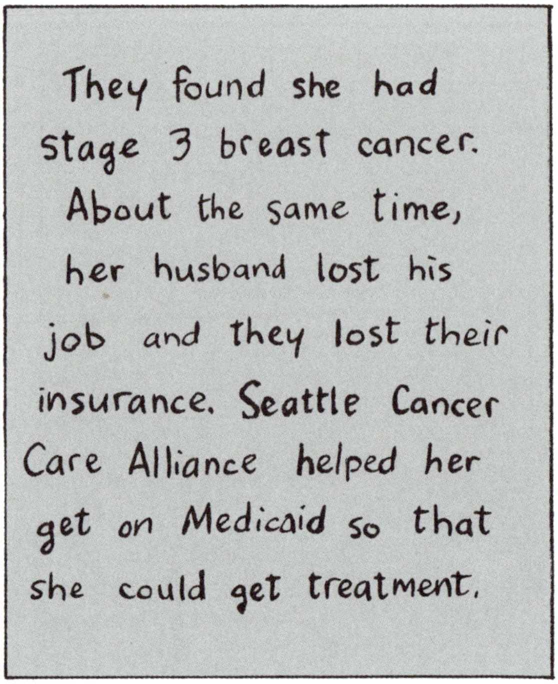
They found she had stage 3 breast cancer. About the same time, her husband lost his job and they lost their insurance. Seattle Cancer Care Alliance helped her get on Medicaid so that she could get treatment.

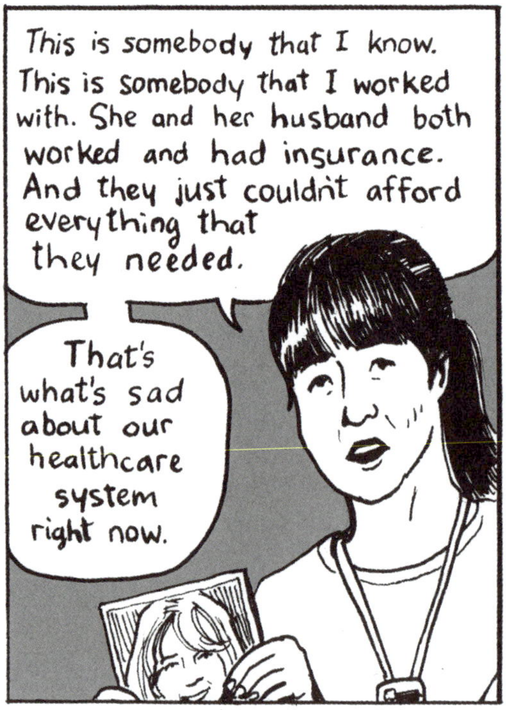
This is somebody that I know. This is somebody that I worked with. She and her husband both worked and had insurance. And they just couldn't afford everything that they needed.
That's what's sad about our healthcare system right now.

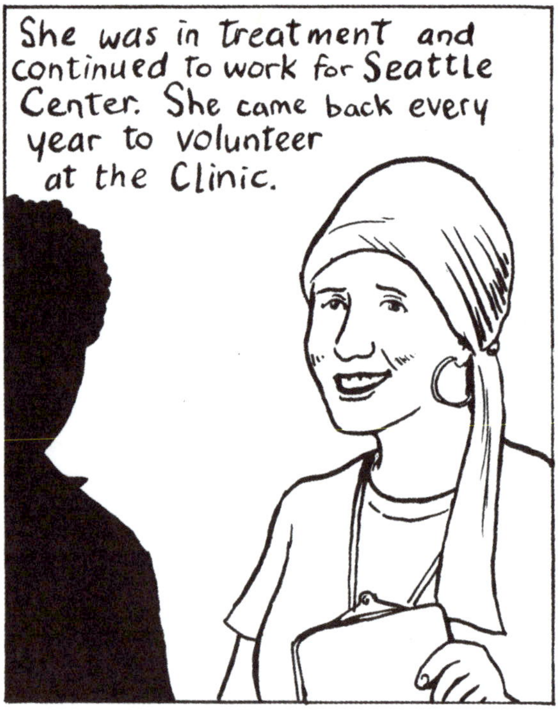
She was in treatment and continued to work for Seattle Center. She came back every year to volunteer at the Clinic.

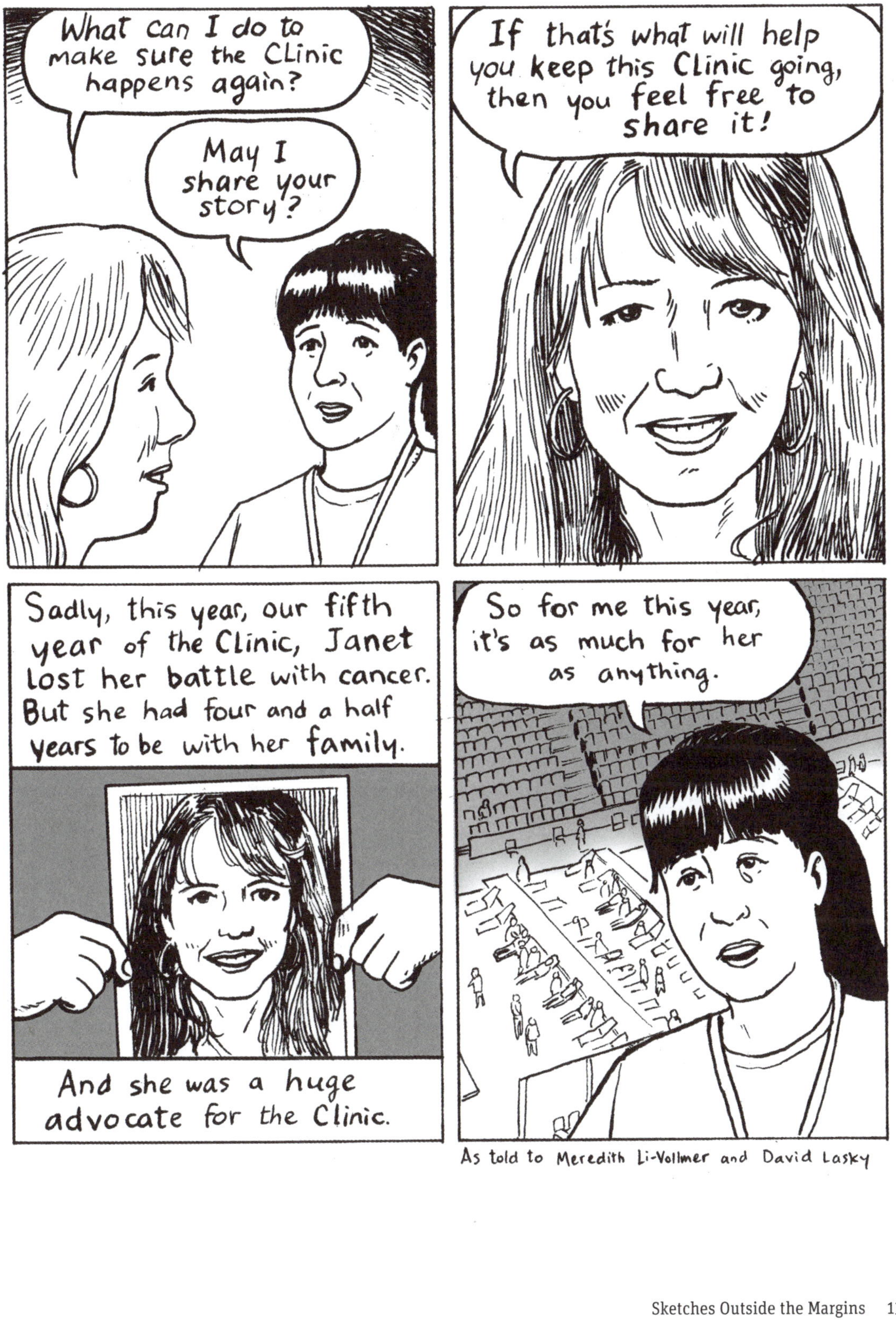
What can I do to make sure the Clinic happens again?
May I share your story?
If that's what will help you keep this Clinic going, then you feel free to share it!
Sadly, this year, our fifth year of the Clinic, Janet lost her battle with cancer. But she had four and a half years to be with her family.
And she was a huge advocate for the Clinic.
So for me this year, it's as much for her as anything.

As told to Meredith Li-Vollmer and David Lasky

EPILOGUE

by Meredith Li-Vollmer

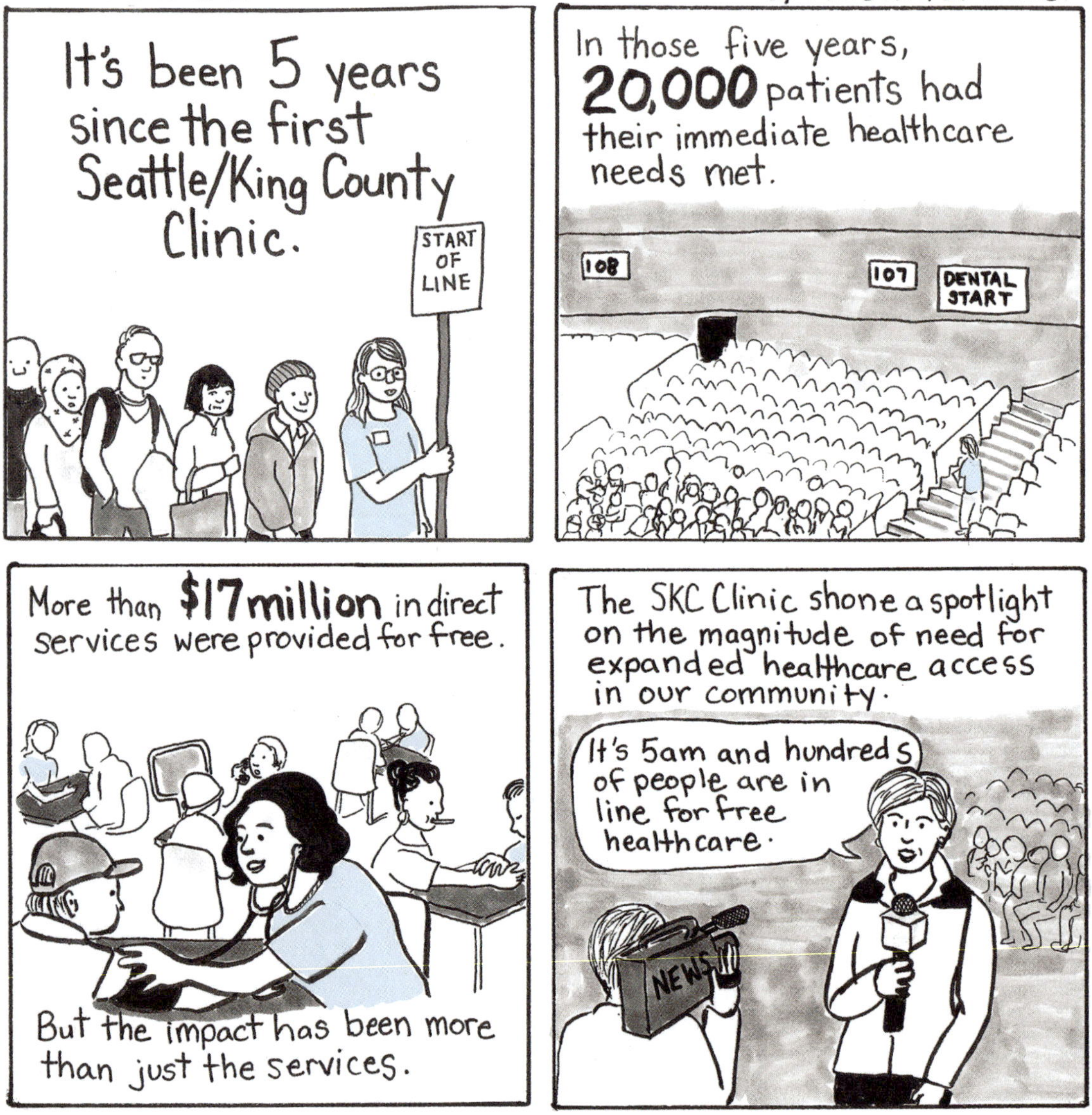
It's been 5 years since the first Seattle/King County Clinic.
START OF LINE
In those five years, 20,000 patients had their immediate healthcare needs met.
108
107
DENTAL START
More than $17 million in direct services were provided for free.
But the impact has been more than just the services.
The SKC Clinic shone a spotlight on the magnitude of need for expanded healthcare access in our community.
It's 5am and hundreds of people are in line for free healthcare.
NEWS

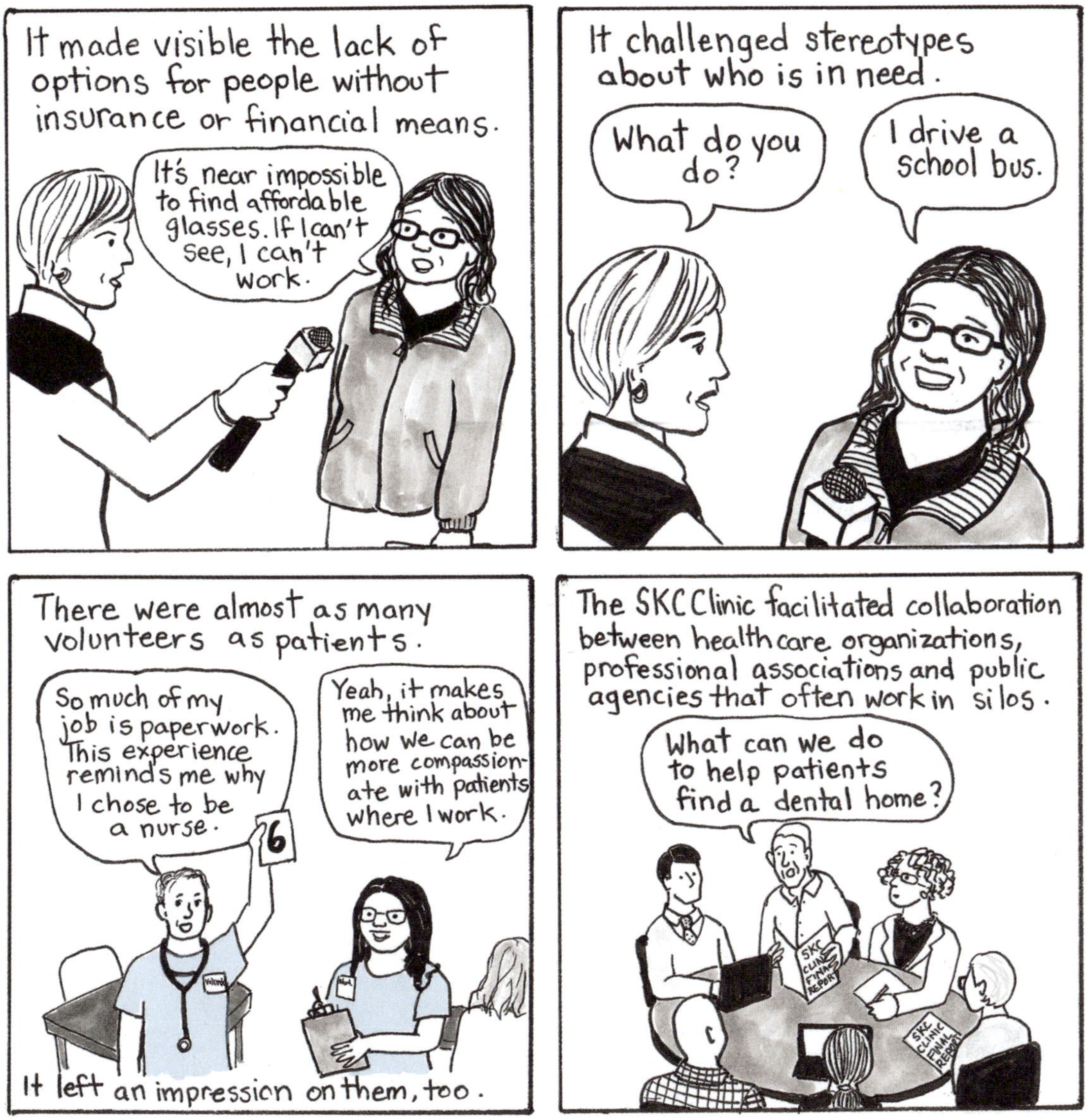
It made visible the lack of options for people without insurance or financial means.
It's near impossible to find affordable glasses. If I can't see, I can't work.
It challenged stereotypes about who is in need.
What do you do?
I drive a school bus.
There were almost as many volunteers as patients.
So much of my job is paperwork. This experience reminds me why I chose to be a nurse.
6
Yeah, it makes me think about how we can be more compassionate with patients where I work.
It left an impression on them, too.
The SKC Clinic facilitated collaboration between health care organizations, professional associations and public agencies that often work in silos.
What can we do to help patients find a dental home?
SKC CLINIC FINAL REPORT

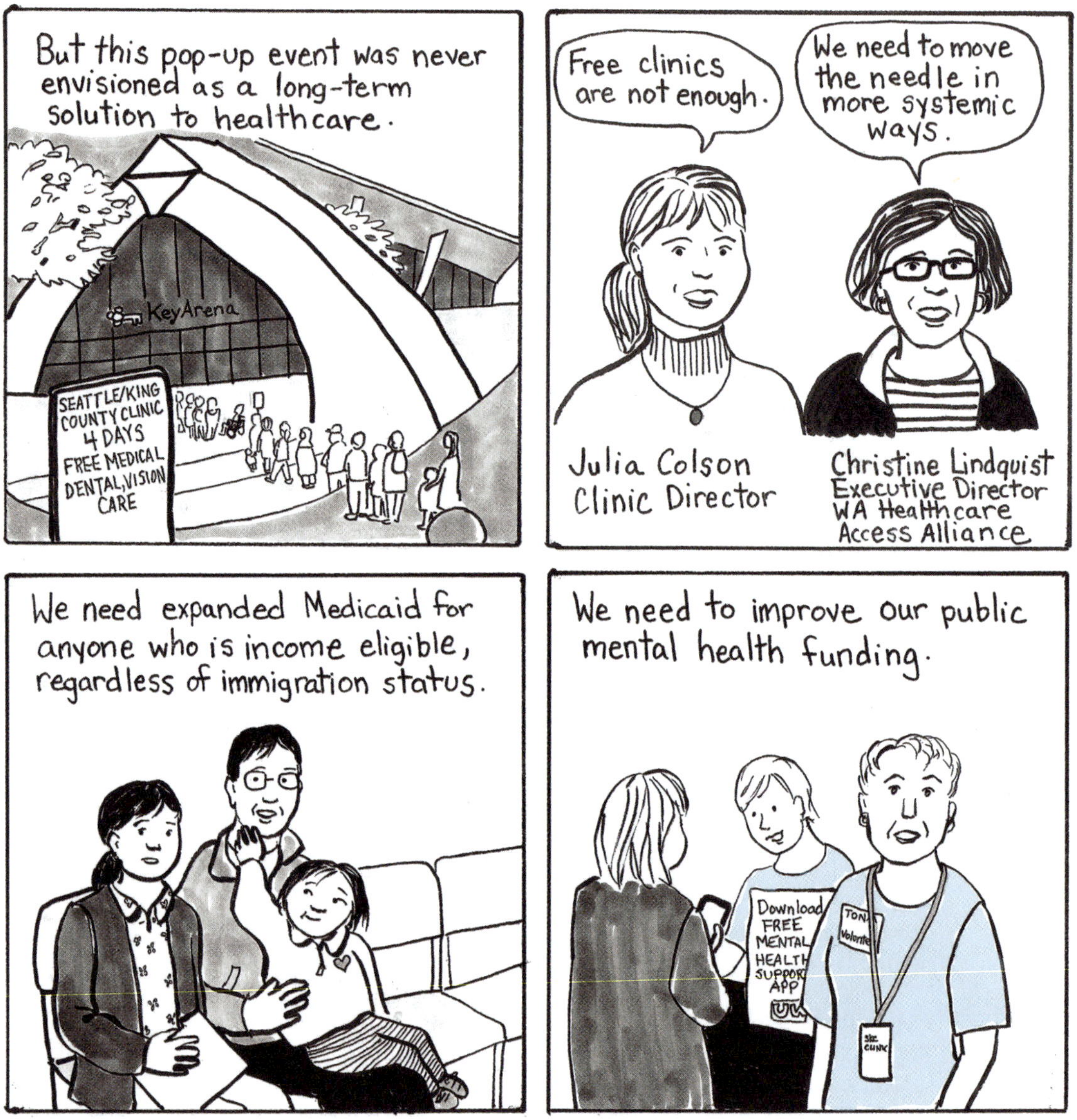
But this pop-up event was never envisioned as a long-term solution to healthcare.
KeyArena
SEATTLE/KING COUNTY CLINIC 4 DAYS FREE MEDICAL DENTAL, VISION CARE
Free clinics are not enough.
We need to move the needle in more systemic ways.
Julia Colson
Clinic Director
Christine Lindquist
Executive Director
WA Healthcare Access Alliance
We need expanded Medicaid for anyone who is income eligible, regardless of immigration status.
We need to improve our public mental health funding.
Download FREE MENTAL HEALTH
APP

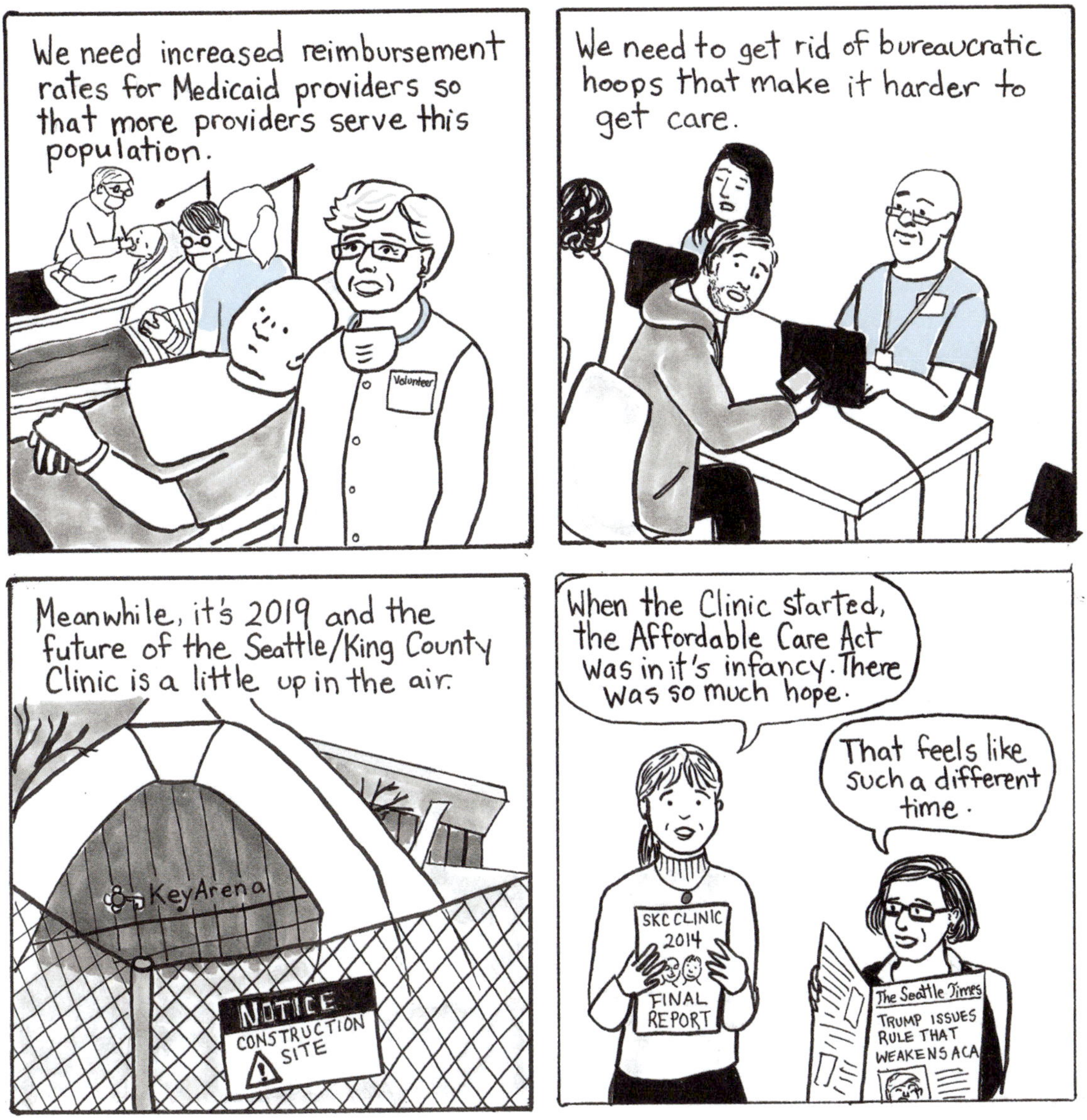
We need increased reimbursement rates for Medicaid providers so that more providers serve this population.
Volunteer
We need to get rid of bureaucratic hoops that make it harder to get care.
Meanwhile, it's 2019 and the future of the Seattle/King County Clinic is a little up in the air.
KeyArena
NOTICE
CONSTRUCTION SITE
When the Clinic started, the Affordable Care Act was in it's infancy. There was so much hope.
That feels like such a different time.
SKC CLINIC 2014 FINAL REPORT
The Seattle Times
TRUMP ISSUES RULE THAT WEAKENS ACA

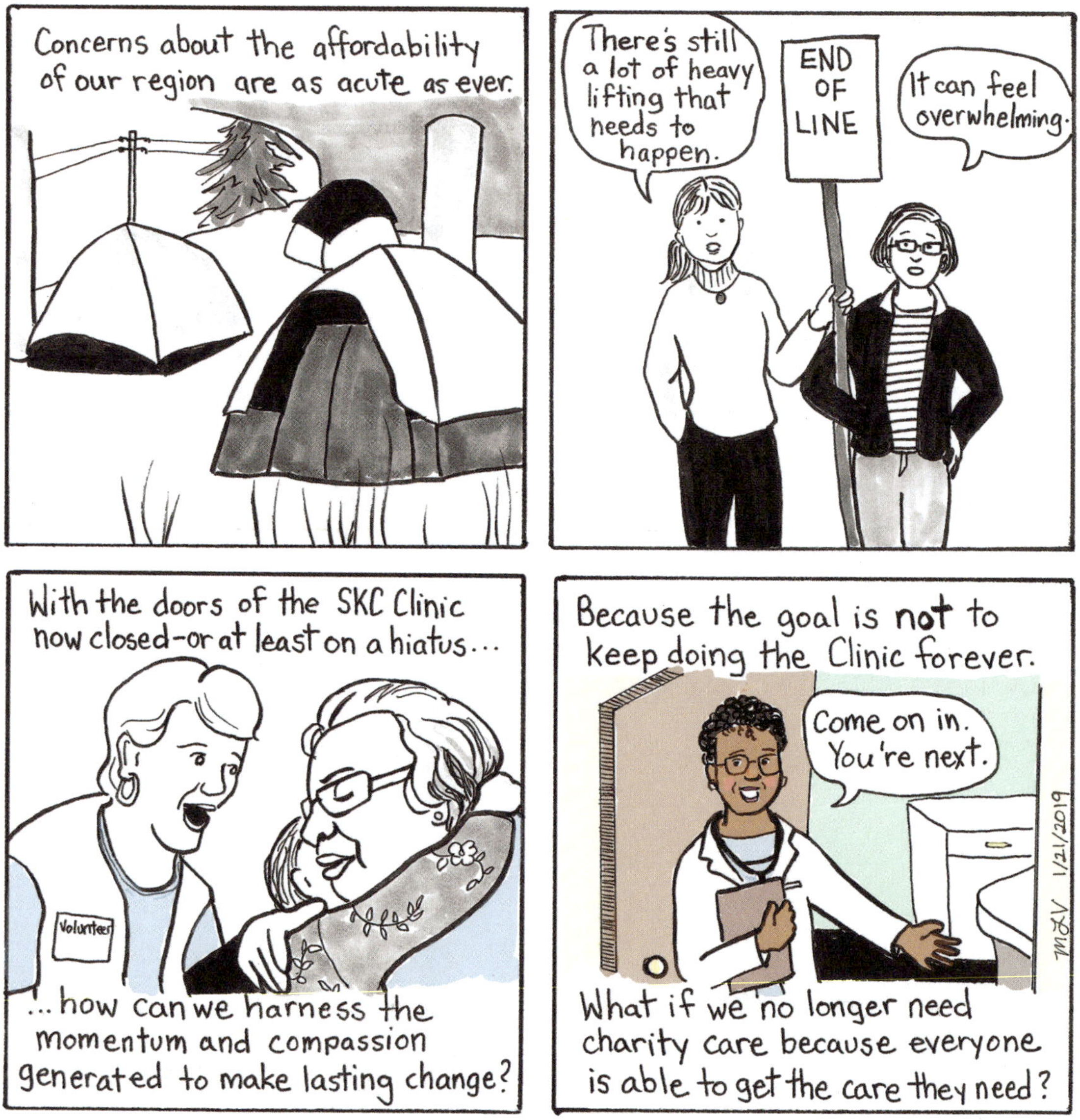
Concerns about the affordability of our region are as acute as ever.
There's still a lot of heavy lifting that needs to happen.
END OF LINE
It can feel overwhelming.
With the doors of the SKC Clinic now closed-or at least on a hiatus...
Volunteer
...how can we harness the momentum and compassion generated to make lasting change?
Because the goal is **not** to keep doing the Clinic forever.
Come on in. You're next.
What if we no longer need charity care because everyone is able to get the care they need?

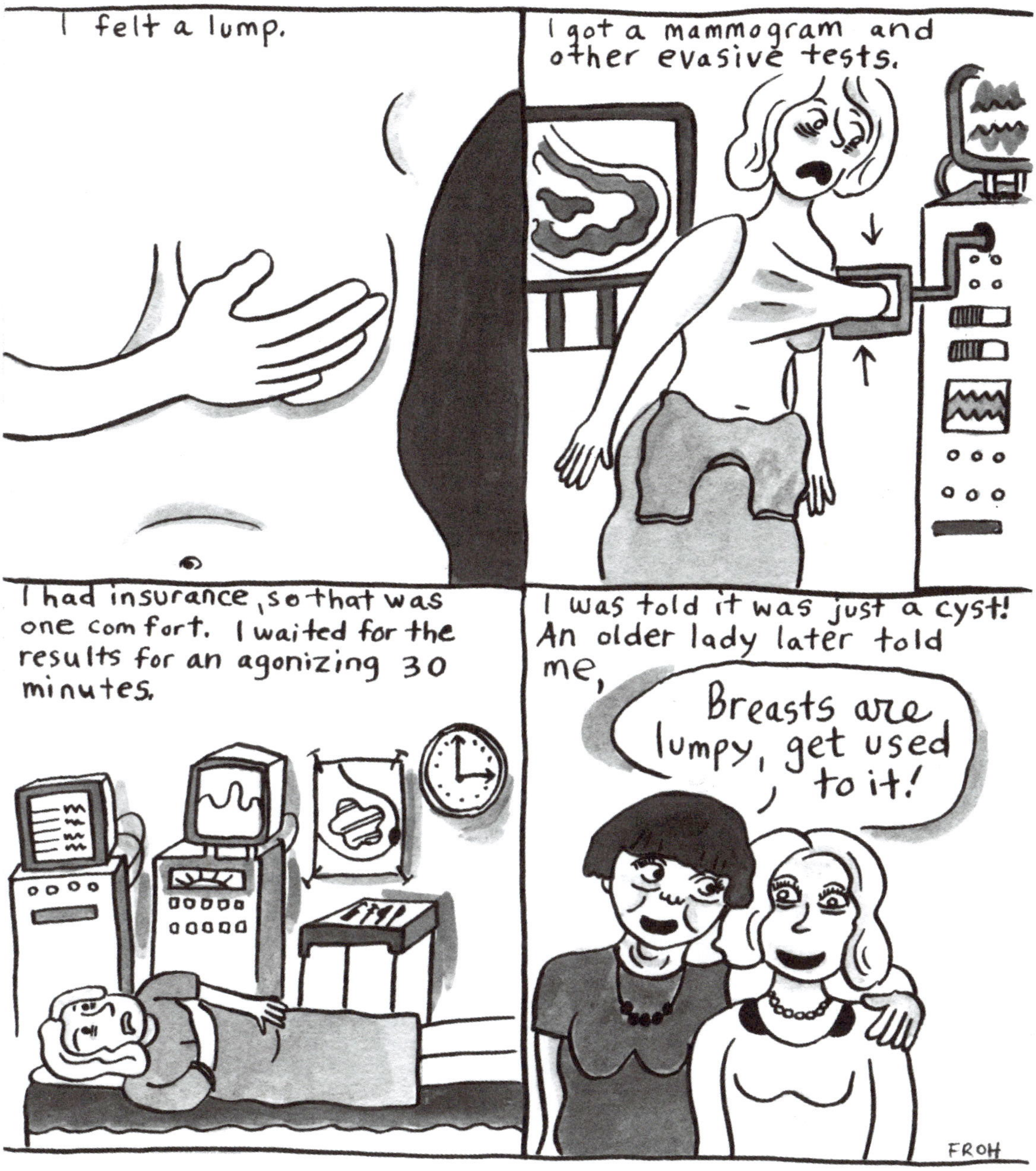
I felt a lump.
I got a mammogram and other evasive tests.
I had insurance, so that was one comfort. I waited for the results for an agonizing 30 minutes.
I was told it was just a cyst! An older lady later told me,
Breasts are lumpy, get used to it!
FROH

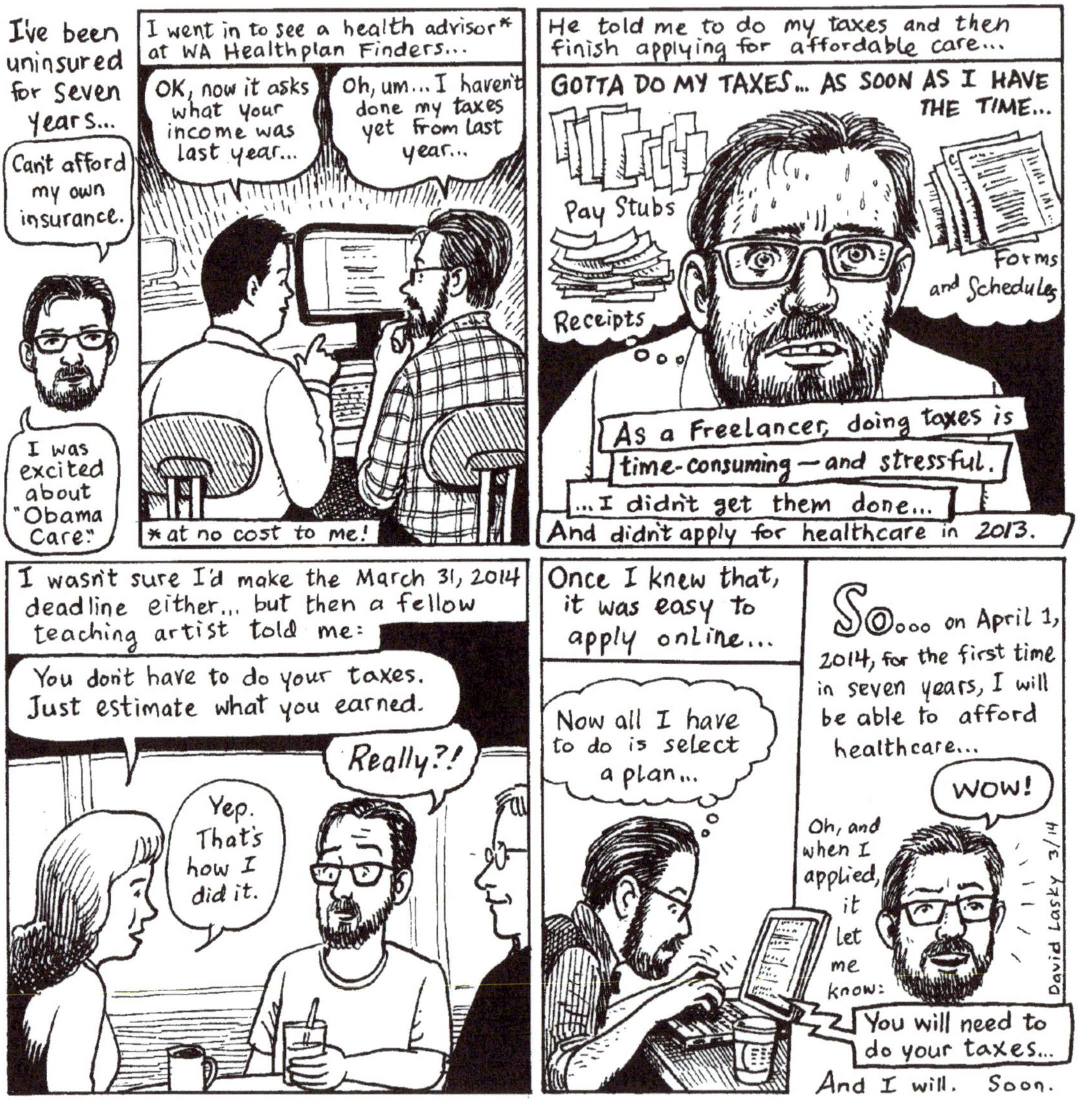

I've been uninsured for seven years...
Can't afford my own insurance.
I was excited about "Obama Care."
I went in to see a health advisor* at WA Healthplan Finders...
OK, now it asks what your income was last year...
Oh, um... I haven't done my taxes yet from last year...
*at no cost to me!
He told me to do my taxes and then finish applying for affordable care...
GOTTA DO MY TAXES... AS SOON AS I HAVE THE TIME...
Pay Stubs
Receipts
Forms and Schedules
As a Freelancer, doing taxes is time-consuming — and stressful.
...I didn't get them done...
And didn't apply for healthcare in 2013.
I wasn't sure I'd make the March 31, 2014 deadline either... but then a fellow teaching artist told me:
You don't have to do your taxes. Just estimate what you earned.
Really?!
Yep. That's how I did it.
Once I knew that, it was easy to apply online...
Now all I have to do is select a plan...
Sooo on April 1, 2014, for the first time in seven years, I will be able to afford healthcare...
WOW!
Oh, and when I applied, it let me know:
You will need to do your taxes...
And I will. Soon.
David Lasky 3/14

Insurance is not assurance.
You will get sick. You may stay sick.
You may die when you don't want to die.
After all, life is made up of lovely who-knows-whats of all shapes and sizes.
STILL- will you please take care? Whatever having CARE means to you —
take care.
m.m.

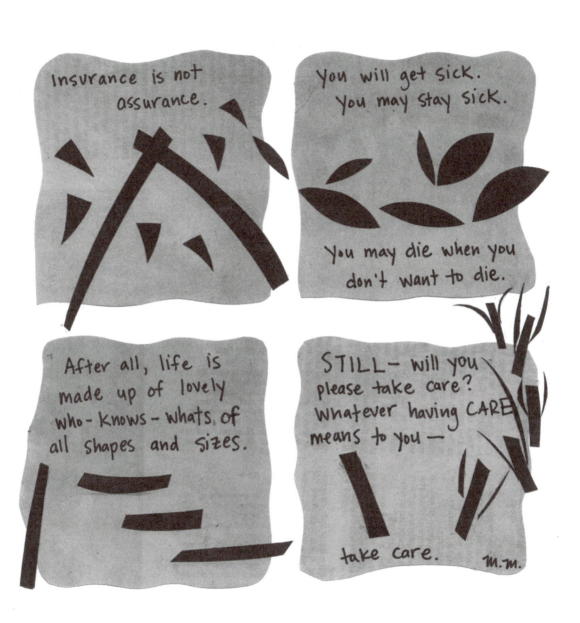

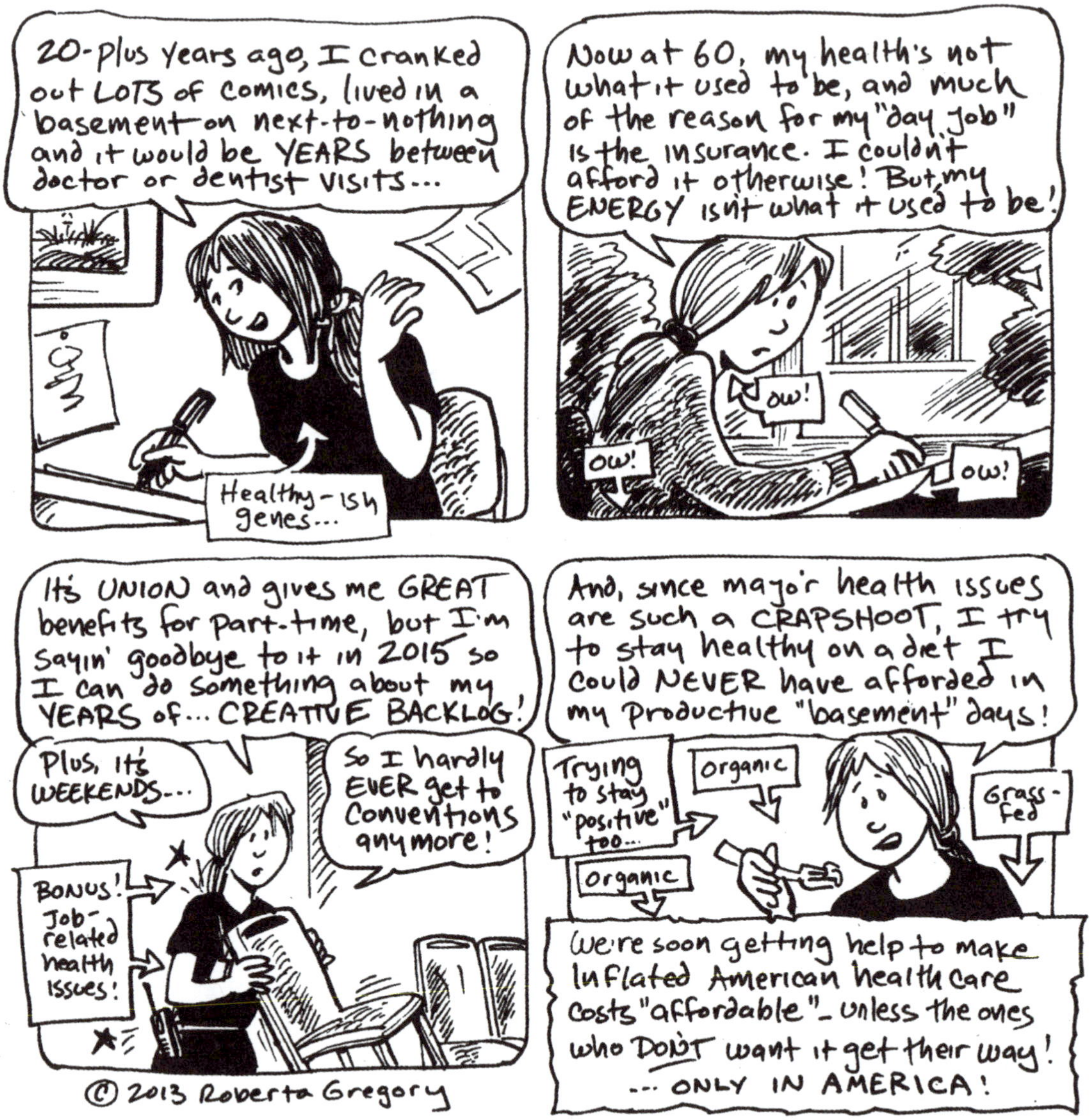
20-plus years ago, I cranked out LOTS of comics, lived in a basement on next-to-nothing and it would be YEARS between doctor or dentist visits...
Healthy-ish genes...
Now at 60, my health's not what it used to be, and much of the reason for my "day job" is the insurance. I couldn't afford it otherwise! But, my ENERGY isn't what it used to be!
OW!
OW!
OW!
It's UNION and gives me GREAT benefits for part-time, but I'm sayin' goodbye to it in 2015 so I can do something about my YEARS of... CREATIVE BACKLOG!
Plus, it's WEEKENDS...
So I hardly EVER get to Conventions anymore!
BONUS! Job-related health issues!
© 2013 Roberta Gregory
And, since major health issues are such a CRAPSHOOT, I try to stay healthy on a diet I could NEVER have afforded in my productive "basement" days!
Trying to stay "positive" too...
organic
organic
Grass-fed
We're soon getting help to make inflated American health care costs "affordable" - unless the ones who DON'T want it get their way! ... ONLY IN AMERICA!

WINDOW

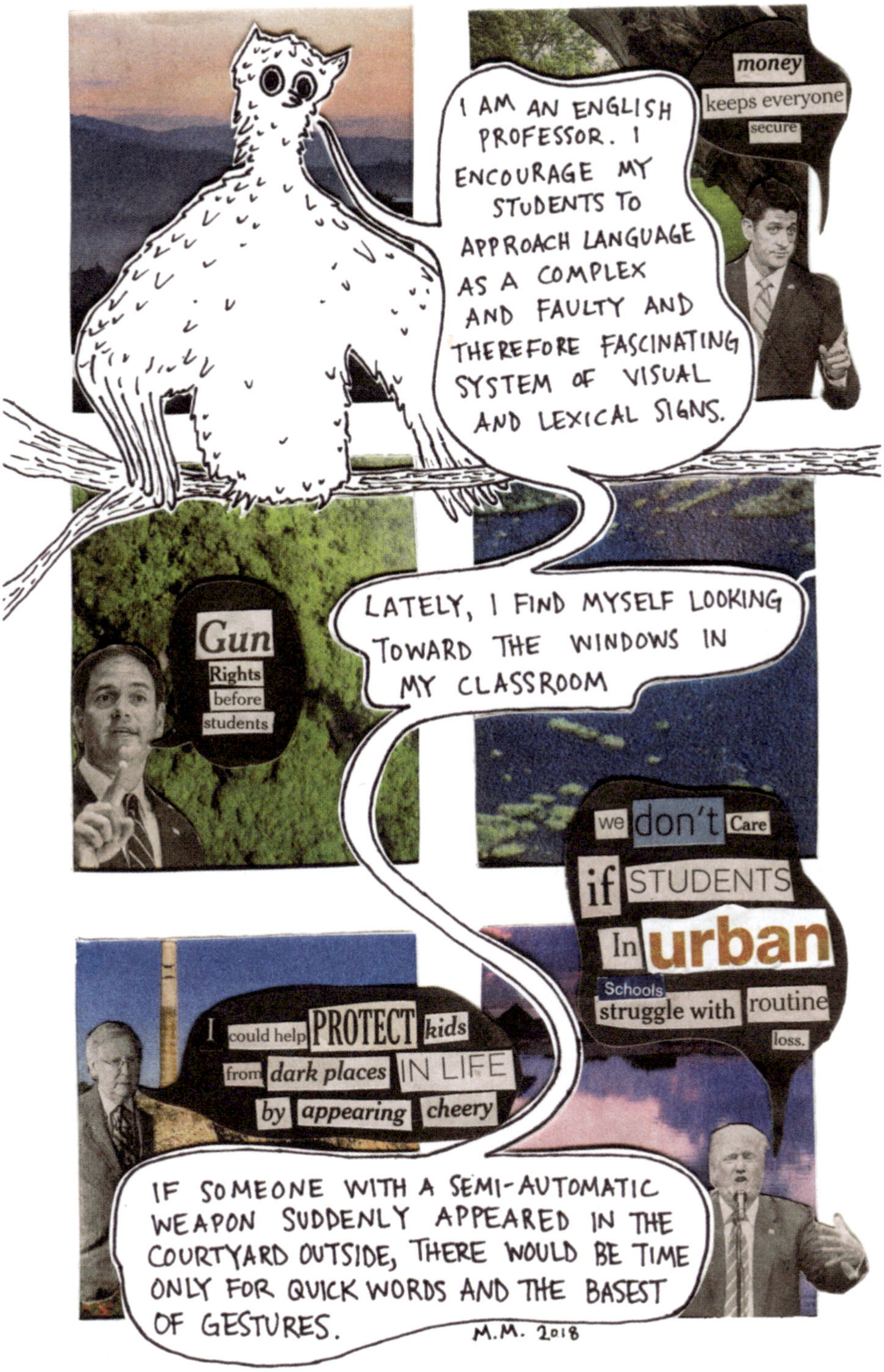
I AM AN ENGLISH PROFESSOR. I ENCOURAGE MY STUDENTS TO APPROACH LANGUAGE AS A COMPLEX AND FAULTY AND THEREFORE FASCINATING SYSTEM OF VISUAL AND LEXICAL SIGNS.
money keeps everyone secure
Gun Rights before students
LATELY, I FIND MYSELF LOOKING TOWARD THE WINDOWS IN MY CLASSROOM
we don't Care if STUDENTS In urban Schools struggle with routine loss.
I could help PROTECT kids from dark places IN LIFE by appearing cheery
IF SOMEONE WITH A SEMI-AUTOMATIC WEAPON SUDDENLY APPEARED IN THE COURTYARD OUTSIDE, THERE WOULD BE TIME ONLY FOR QUICK WORDS AND THE BASEST OF GESTURES.
M.M. 2018

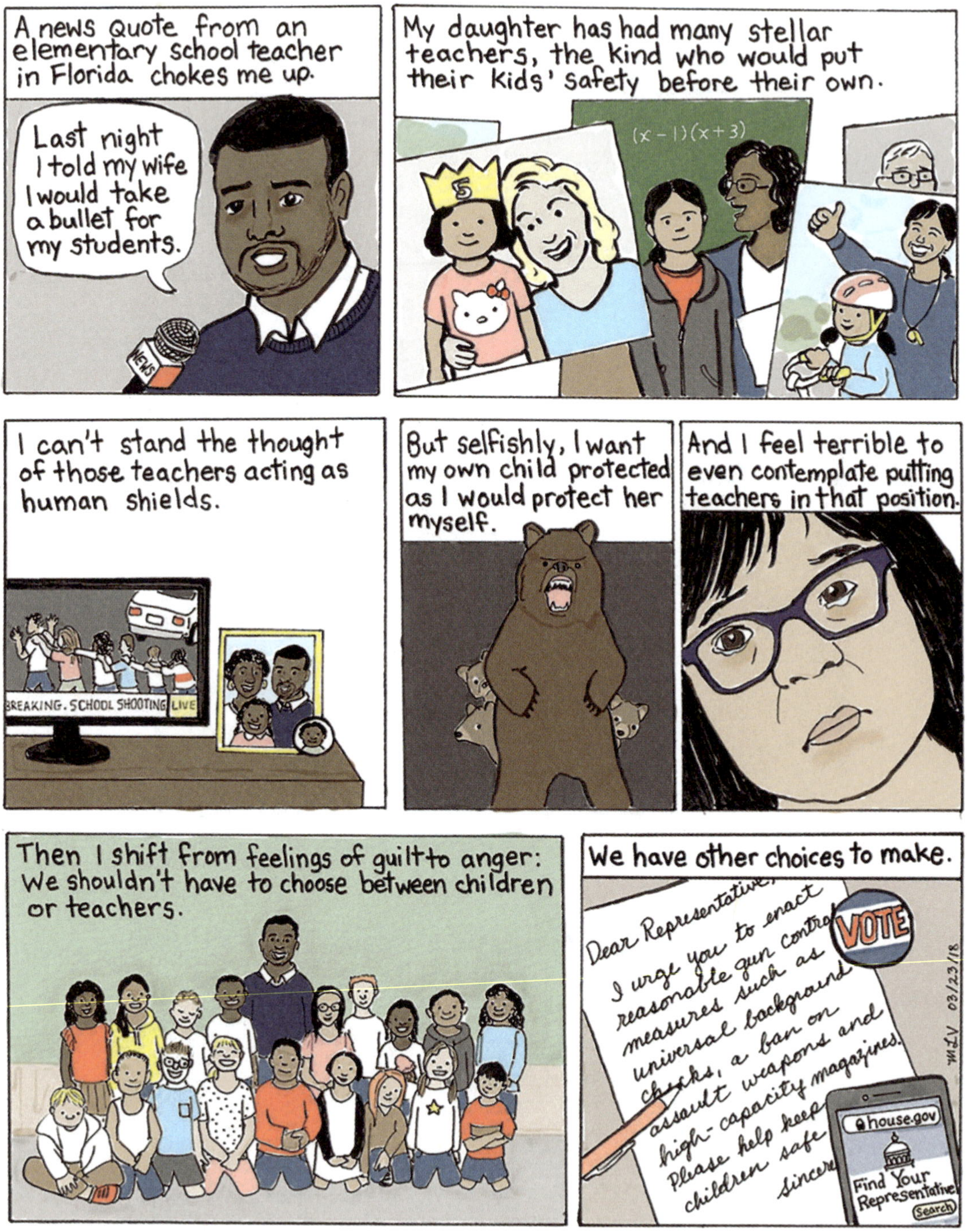

A news quote from an elementary school teacher in Florida chokes me up.
Last night I told my wife I would take a bullet for my students.
NEWS
My daughter has had many stellar teachers, the kind who would put their kids' safety before their own.
5
(x − 1)(x + 3)
I can't stand the thought of those teachers acting as human shields.
BREAKING. SCHOOL SHOOTING LIVE
But selfishly, I want my own child protected as I would protect her myself.
And I feel terrible to even contemplate putting teachers in that position.
Then I shift from feelings of guilt to anger: We shouldn't have to choose between children or teachers.
We have other choices to make.
Dear Representative,
I urge you to enact reasonable gun
measures such as universal background checks, a ban on assault weapons and high-capacity magazines.
Please help keep children safe
VOTE
house.gov
Find Your Representative
Search
MLV 03/23/18

DRILLED by ellen forney

FEB. 2018. I ASKED THE DIRECTOR OF COLLEGE MENTAL HEALTH SERVICES FOR ADVICE ON LEADING A CLASSROOM DISCUSSION ON PARKLAND.

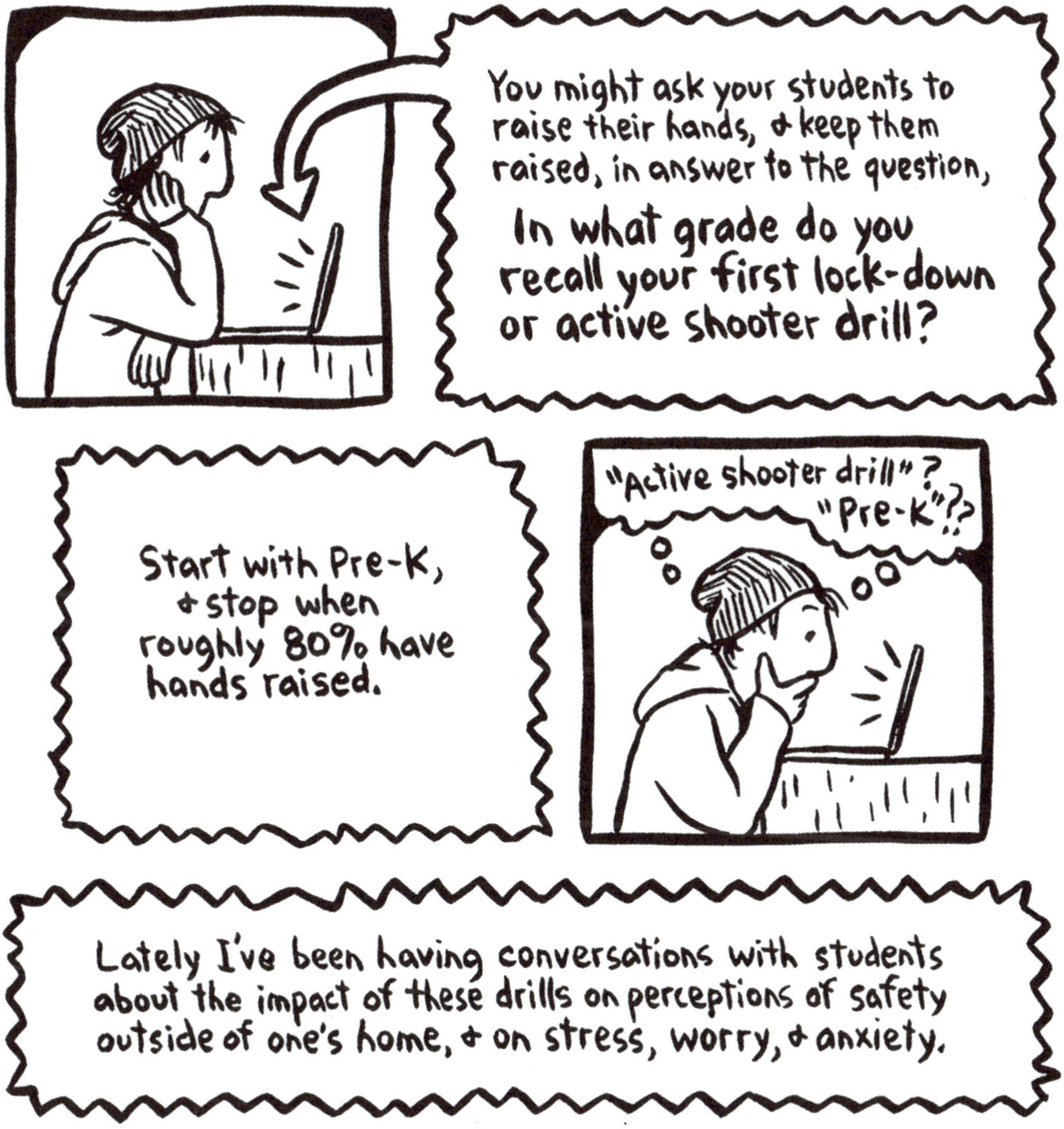
You might ask your students to raise their hands, & keep them raised, in answer to the question,
In what grade do you recall your first lock-down or active shooter drill?
Start with Pre-K, & stop when roughly 80% have hands raised.
"Active shooter drill"? "Pre-K"??
Lately I've been having conversations with students about the impact of these drills on perceptions of safety outside of one's home, & on stress, worry, & anxiety.

How many of you had active shooter drills at school?

Wait-- Pre-K, 80%...
You mean, lock-downs?
Isn't that kind of the same thing?
How many of you have had lock-downs in school?

plop!

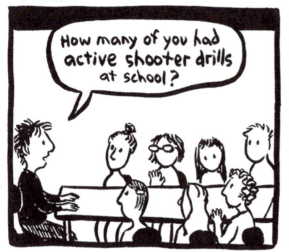

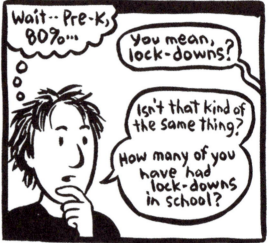

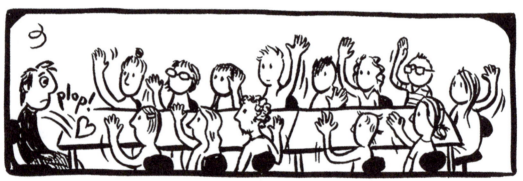

IT WAS AS IF I'D ASKED IF THEY EVER HAD FIRE DRILLS, OR POP QUIZZES, OR BAD CAFETERIA FOOD.

I HAD A WAVE OF IRRATIONAL PROTECTIVENESS THAT LASTED FOR DAYS.

My little lambs!
How we've failed them!

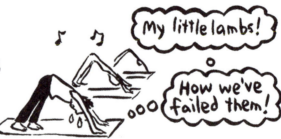

SO MANY OF THEM ARE ON MEDS FOR ANXIETY.

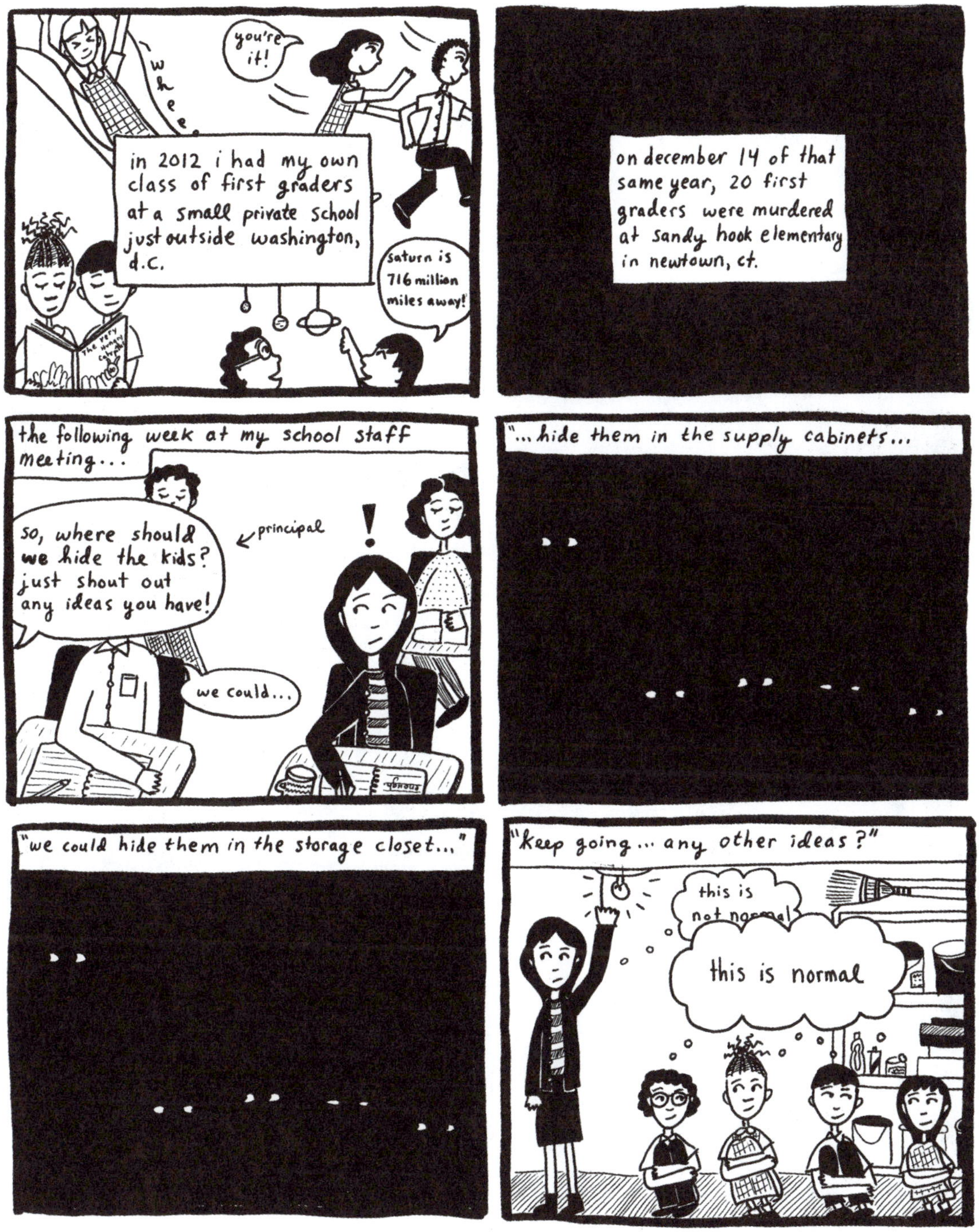
whee
you're it!
in 2012 i had my own class of first graders at a small private school just outside washington, d.c.
saturn is 716 million miles away!
on december 14 of that same year, 20 first graders were murdered at sandy hook elementary in newtown, ct.
the following week at my school staff meeting...
so, where should we hide the kids? just shout out any ideas you have!
principal
!
we could...
"...hide them in the supply cabinets...
"we could hide them in the storage closet..."
"keep going... any other ideas?"
this is not normal
this is normal

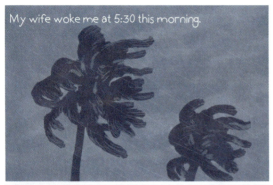

My wife woke me at 5:30 this morning.

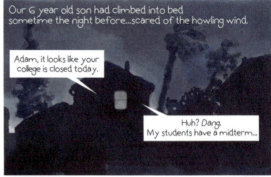

Our 6 year old son had climbed into bed sometime the night before...scared of the howling wind.

Adam, it looks like your college is closed today.

Huh? Dang. My students have a midterm...

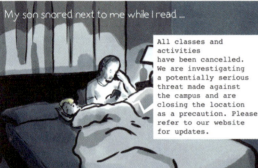

My son snored next to me while I read ...

All classes and activities have been cancelled. We are investigating a potentially serious threat made against the campus and are closing the location as a precaution. Please refer to our website for updates.

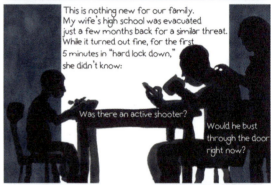

This is nothing new for our family. My wife's high school was evacuated just a few months back for a similar threat. While it turned out fine, for the first 5 minutes in "hard lock down," she didn't know:

Was there an active shooter?

Would he bust through the door right now?

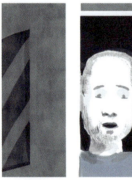

Bye honey!

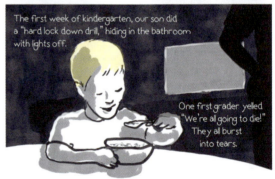

The first week of kindergarten, our son did a "hard lock down drill," hiding in the bathroom with lights off.

One first grader yelled "We're all going to die!" They all burst into tears.

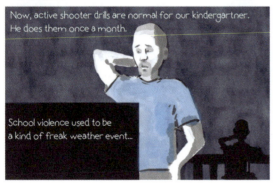

Now, active shooter drills are normal for our kindergartner. He does them once a month.

School violence used to be a kind of freak weather event...

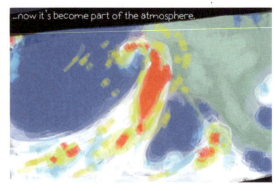

...now it's become part of the atmosphere.

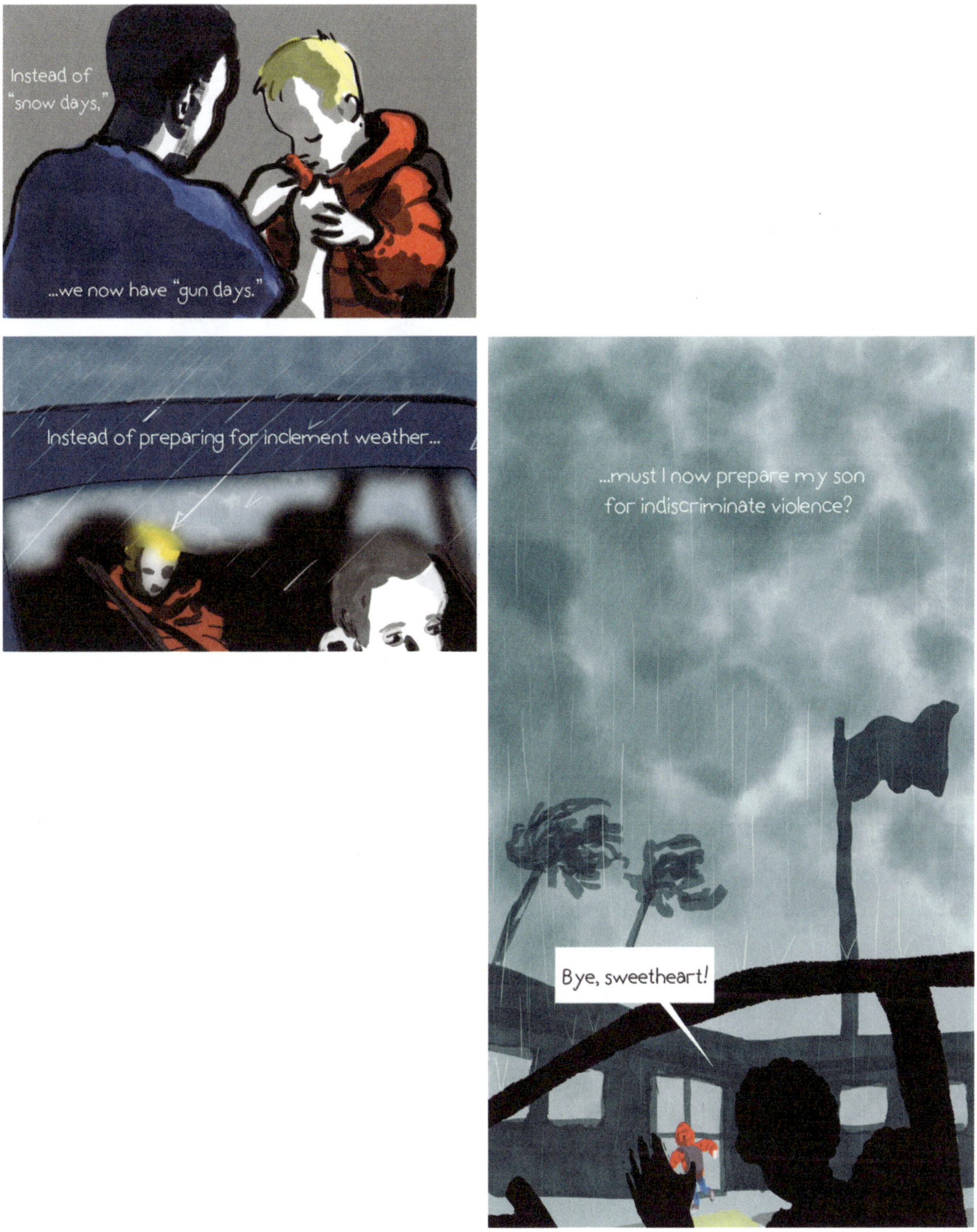
Instead of "snow days,"
...we now have "gun days."
Instead of preparing for inclement weather...
...must I now prepare my son for indiscriminate violence?
Bye, sweetheart!

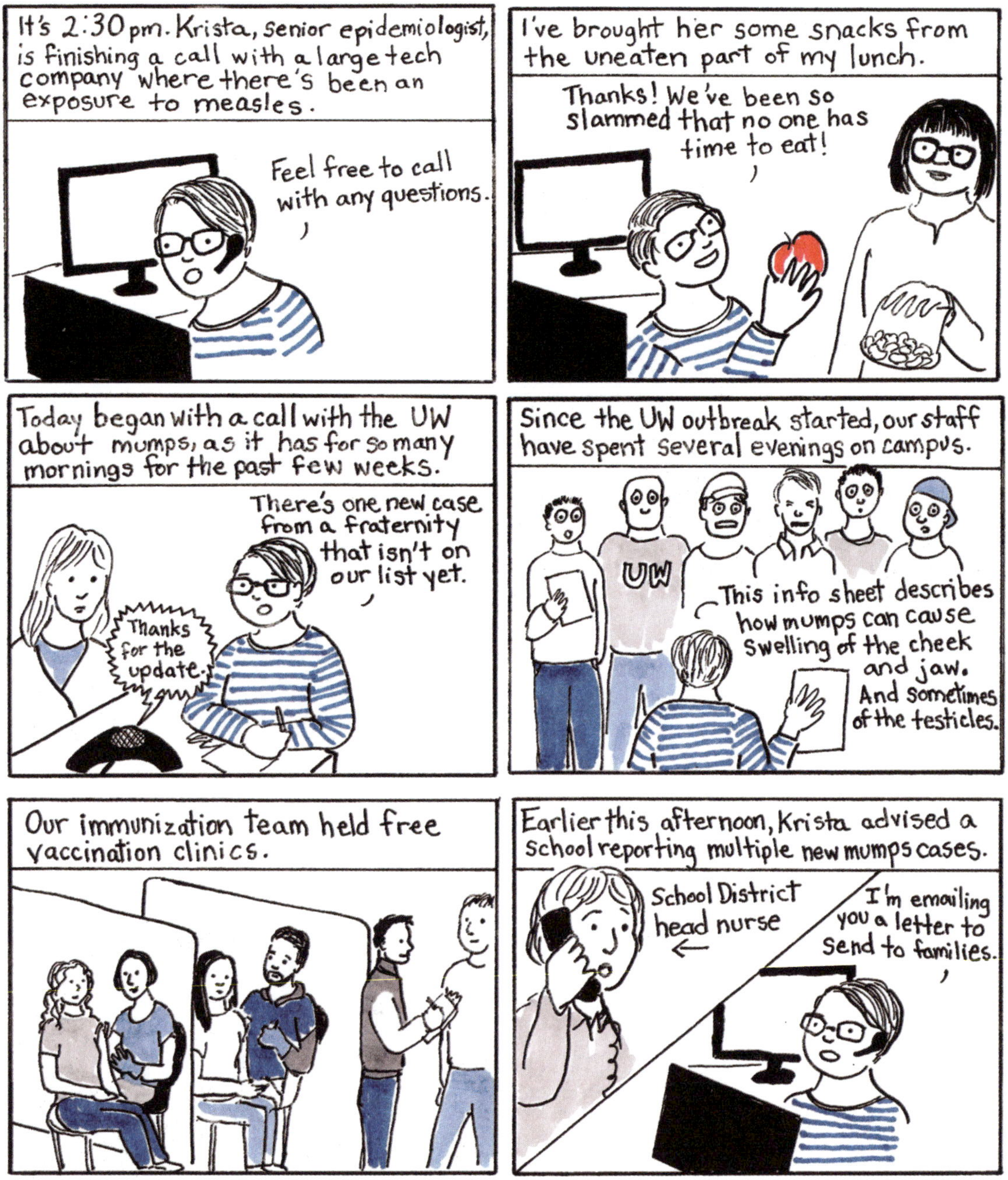
It's 2:30 pm. Krista, senior epidemiologist, is finishing a call with a large tech company where there's been an exposure to measles.
Feel free to call with any questions.
I've brought her some snacks from the uneaten part of my lunch.
Thanks! We've been so slammed that no one has time to eat!
Today began with a call with the UW about mumps, as it has for so many mornings for the past few weeks.
There's one new case from a fraternity that isn't on our list yet.
Thanks for the update.
Since the UW outbreak started, our staff have spent several evenings on campus.
UW
This info sheet describes how mumps can cause swelling of the cheek and jaw. And sometimes of the testicles.
Our immunization team held free vaccination clinics.
Earlier this afternoon, Krista advised a school reporting multiple new mumps cases.
School District head nurse ←
I'm emailing you a letter to send to families.

Every nurse and disease investigator is busy working on a case as I walk past their cubicles:

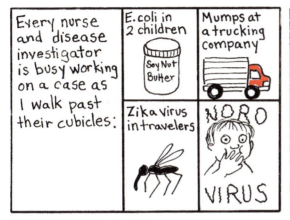

E. coli in 2 children

Soy Nut Butter

Mumps at a trucking company

Zika virus in travelers

NORO VIRUS

Staff take turns being on-call so someone can start a disease investigation 24/7.

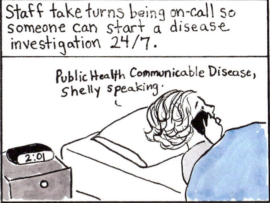

Public Health Communicable Disease, Shelly speaking.

2:01

Others in our department play support roles, like communications.

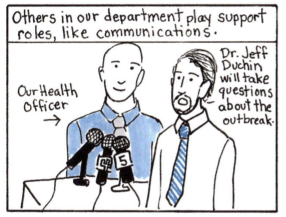

Our Health Officer →

Dr. Jeff Duchin will take questions about the outbreak.

5

...and our emergency preparedness unit.

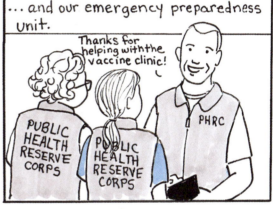

Thanks for helping with the vaccine clinic!

PUBLIC HEALTH RESERVE CORPS

PUBLIC HEALTH RESERVE CORPS

PHRC

This is Dr. Meagan Kay. She's a medical epidemiologist and she supervises the disease investigation group.

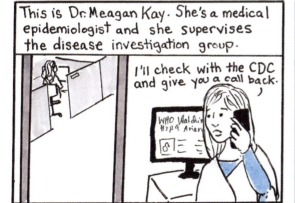

I'll check with the CDC and give you a call back.

WHO Watching H7N9 Avian

Earlier this week she met with neighbors of a King County resident who died from hantavirus to address their concerns.

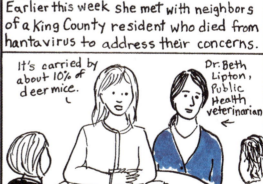

It's carried by about 10% of deer mice.

Dr. Beth Lipton, Public Health veterinarian ←

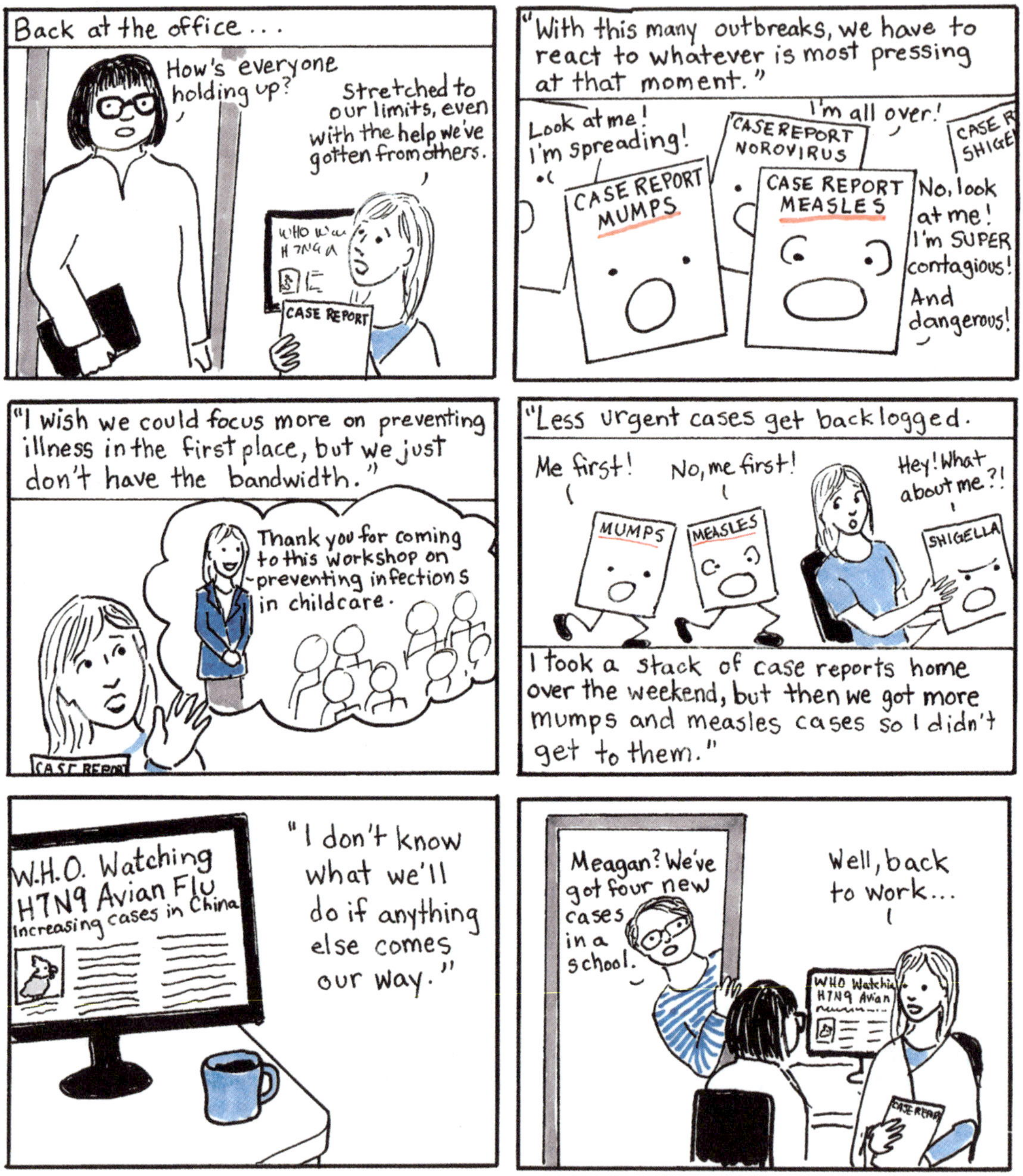
Back at the office . . .
How's everyone holding up?
Stretched to our limits, even with the help we've gotten from others.
CASE REPORT
"With this many outbreaks, we have to react to whatever is most pressing at that moment."
Look at me! I'm spreading!
I'm all over!
CASE REPORT NOROVIRUS
CASE REPORT MUMPS
CASE REPORT MEASLES
No, look at me! I'm SUPER contagious!
And dangerous!
"I wish we could focus more on preventing illness in the first place, but we just don't have the bandwidth."
Thank you for coming to this workshop on preventing infections in childcare.
"Less urgent cases get backlogged.
Me first!
No, me first!
Hey! What about me?!
MUMPS
MEASLES
SHIGELLA
I took a stack of case reports home over the weekend, but then we got more mumps and measles cases so I didn't get to them."
W.H.O. Watching H7N9 Avian Flu
Increasing cases in China
"I don't know what we'll do if anything else comes our way."
Meagan? We've got four new cases in a school.
Well, back to work . . .

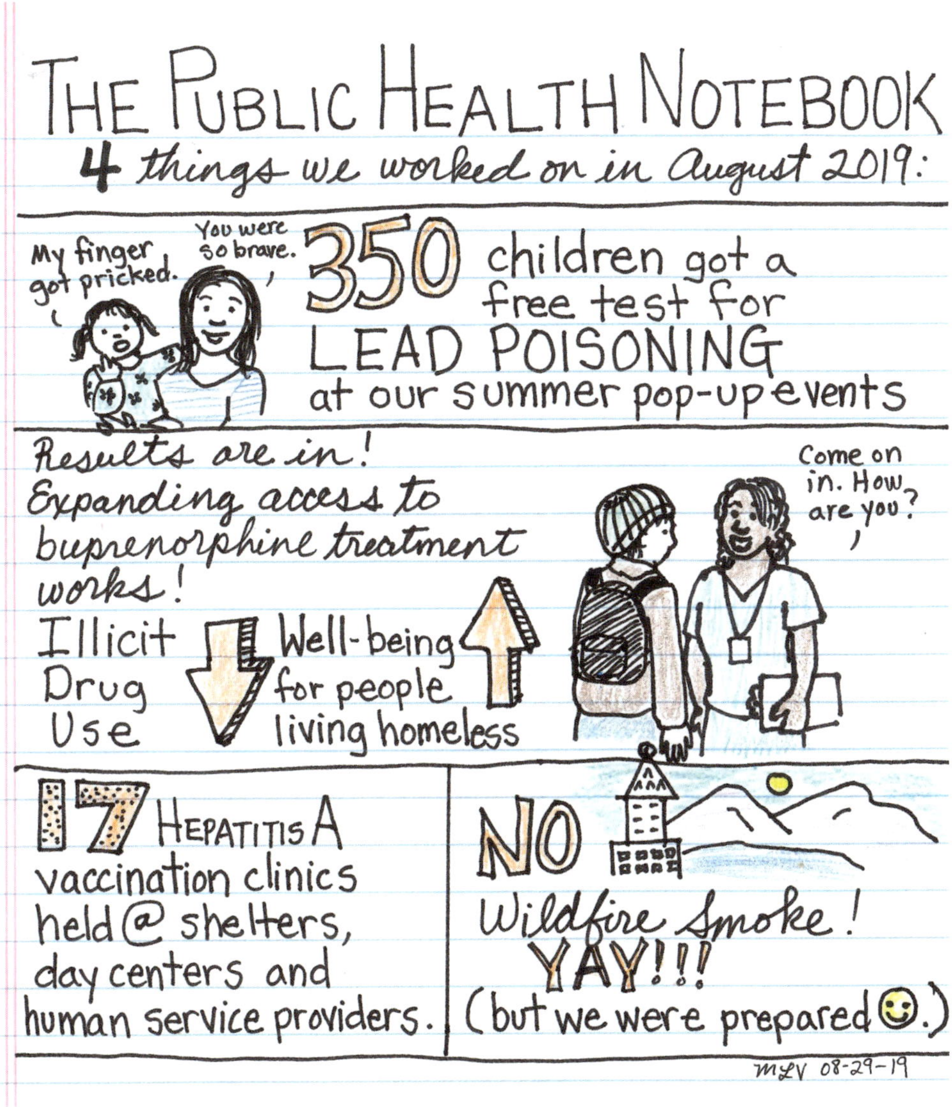

THE PUBLIC HEALTH NOTEBOOK
4 things we worked on in August 2019:
My finger got pricked.
You were so brave.
350 children got a free test for LEAD POISONING at our summer pop-up events
Results are in! Expanding access to buprenorphine treatment works!
Come on in. How are you?
Illicit Drug Use
Well-being for people living homeless
17 HEPATITIS A vaccination clinics held @ shelters, day centers and human service providers.
NO Wildfire Smoke! YAY!!!
(but we were prepared.)
MLV 08-29-19

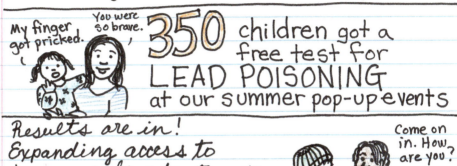

Discussion

The central mission of public health is to improve health outcomes for communities and reduce health disparities. But the systemic and social issues at the heart of this work—those that determine the health and well-being of communities and individuals—are complex to communicate. Public health professionals need to engage people who don't yet share our passion to support the policy and systemic changes we need. As a visually arresting, empathy-building storytelling medium, comics can help us.

Comics Can Communicate About Tough Topics

Communication about the social determinants of health frequently veers toward wonky explanations and big-picture discussions of impersonal structural issues like housing, city planning, and public policy. And talking about the social determinants of health means talking about institutional oppressions such as income inequality and racism, topics that are intimidating or uncomfortable for many audiences. How do you begin the discussion if some people avoid the topic?

Discussions at the big-picture level may not connect with wide audiences, but down at the ground level are stories about real people. Their health is defined by the resources for healthy living that are available (or absent) in their neighborhoods, the prospects they have for education and employment, and the opportunities or barriers created by the policies at play where they live. The focus of public health is moving beyond the level of individual choices; for instance, individuals should not be held solely responsible for their nutritional choices when income disparity, food deserts in their neighborhoods, and the proliferation of cheap fast-food businesses are all part of the equation. Using comics, we can tell individual stories that shed light on these larger systemic issues without reducing the issues to matters of individual-level responsibility.

The narrative and sequential nature of comics are made for telling stories, and the images can provide visual context for complex issues while keeping people front and center. Comics can make upstream issues more human. Public policy becomes more concrete and emotionally urgent when readers can connect it to a person whose face is right in front of them.

Comics may also engage people more deeply in the complexity of multifaceted public health issues because, as medical anthropologist Stacy Pigg explains, they "communicate not through propositional statements, but through display."[1] Active cognitive involvement is required to make meaning of the layered visual elements in narrative comics. Moreover, the empathetic nature of comics creates possibilities for readers to explore new or multiple perspectives. Like other narrative forms, comics embody feelings, motives, ideas, and perspectives of the characters shown. But comics display these stories with visual specificity and multiple modes of evoking the senses, uniquely inviting readers to project themselves into the situation. Pigg also argues that context awareness is inherent in comics, as readers make sense of the visual descriptions and also interpret what is left out of the comics panels.[2] Focused attention to the contextual elements and juxtapositions of different contexts allows the context of the social relationships, situation, and places to come to the foreground. For communications about population health issues, this attention to context has powerful possibilities.

Sketches Outside the Margins: Patient Stories from a Pop-Up Clinic

The comics in this chapter from the Seattle / King County Clinic demonstrate how to connect human stories to public policy. The Seattle / King County Clinic is a giant event held for four days every year. A collective effort by more than one hundred local organizations and legions of volunteers, it offers free medical, dental, and vision care to anyone in need. Several thousand people receive care over the four days, lining up for hours and even overnight at the clinic site at the Seattle Center (home of the Space Needle, a professional hockey/basketball arena, and many performing arts venues).

Julia Colson, director of the Seattle / King County Clinic, wanted to engage policy makers and members of the public in larger conversations about addressing the gaps in the health care system that drive so many people to the clinic. How could we leverage the altruistic energy and attention garnered by the clinic, Colson asked, to advocate for changes that would end the need for mass-scale charity care? We agreed that telling the stories of the patients through comics could put a human face on the issues and potentially provide an entry point for conversations about health care access.

With the support of Colson and the Seattle Center Foundation, I assembled a dream team of cartoonists for a comics journalism project. The team talked to patients on the floor of the giant clinic, with the directive to capture the diversity of people who sought care, why they came to the clinic, and what barriers they faced getting health care elsewhere. Working in the comics medium allowed us to offer patients the option to change their names or request alterations in the details of their appearances so that their privacy could be preserved while we presented stories in their own words. Over the three years of the project, we completed more than seventy short comics telling patient and volunteer stories as well as a few longer pieces about the clinic itself, such as Eroyn Franklin's "Can Free Pop-Up Clinics Save American Healthcare?," which was first published on the online comics site *The Nib*.

Putting a Human Face on Health Care Access

One of the successes of this project was in the sheer number of patient stories we could share, only some of which are included in this chapter. Taken together, they illustrate the enormous need for low-cost health care (even in an affluent area like Seattle) and the wide range of people who struggle to get the care they need. The comics included stories about patients who had experienced homelessness, immigrants who didn't qualify for health insurance under the Affordable Care Act (ACA), and people who were unemployed. These are the kinds of patients that the media and political rhetoric often meld into a faceless mass. The artists were able to provide more of the context of these individuals' circumstances, even in just four to six panels, and once illustrated, people in need became real and relatable.

There were also numerous stories about people whose struggles with health care are common but not always in the spotlight. When we started this project, we wanted to show that despite the wider availability of health coverage under the ACA, many gaps still existed that made health care out of reach. In the last two years of the project, after the Trump administration came into power, these gaps in health care access were compounded by fear that any gains made by the ACA would fall away entirely.

Some of the comics draw attention to the types of patients who aren't as closely associated with charity health care, such as families with children. Other comics in the collection shine light on people who are employed but who don't get health insurance from their employers, who are underinsured, or who struggle to pay their high premiums.

Comics Encourage Empathy and Give Voice

Meeting these individual patients through the comics, and hearing about their health care interactions in their own words, also encourages readers to connect with what each patient has been through. In the comics, you see the individuals who struggle to get health care: the fatigue in their bodies from waiting in lines, the gratitude in their faces after they've received long put-off care, the eye contact with you—the reader—as they share their hardships and their concerns about the future of health care. The comic panels help promote empathy as we meet the patients' family members, witness what brought them to the clinic, and catch glimpses of their lives outside the clinic.

We hoped that the empathy engendered by the medium would help readers open up to the perspectives of the patients, especially by spotlighting voices that often are left out of discussions about health care policy. For "Mixed Blessing," through a Spanish interpreter, I interviewed an extended family of immigrants at the 2018 Seattle / King County Clinic, which was held in the same month during which the Trump administration was proposing to deny entry or green cards to immigrants who used government services, including Medicaid. The parents in the family asked me to tell people about how hardworking immigrants are deserving of health coverage; they also raised questions about how health care resources are prioritized for emergency care rather than preventive care. I added details about this family—such as the restlessness of the children, who had been waiting many hours—to try to make them relatable and share the real story of people in our community who experience hardships because of inadequate health care policy.

Sparking Conversation

The intention of the *Sketches from Outside the Margins* project was to stimulate conversation about the struggles that many people face with health care and the need for solutions, so the team of artists and the organizers of the clinic found multiple avenues to make the comics publicly visible. We got the comics placed in local publications, such as the local alternative weeklies *The Stranger* and *Real Change*, and ethnic community media, like the *International Examiner*. Nationally, they were published online on *The Nib* and *Illustrated PEN*. We also exhibited the comics at the Seattle Public Library and at local eateries and businesses.

Clinic director Julia Colson and I particularly wanted to get the stories in front of people with the power to make decisions about health care policy. With funding from the Seattle Center Foundation, we sent copies of the *Sketches Outside the Margins* anthology to the executives of the more than one hundred organizations that participate in the clinic, including many of the major health care systems and medical associations in our region. Nearly every elected official representing Seattle and the surrounding area received an anthology, including Seattle's mayor and city council members, the King County Board of Health, and the congressional delegation. Copies of the anthology were placed in the waiting room for the regents of the University of Washington, in the University's special collections and health sciences libraries, and delivered to UW's schools of dentistry, public health, and medicine. An exhibit of the comics was even displayed at a regional medical conference, along with Post-it Notes for attendees to share and discuss their reactions.

Personal stories often have the greatest impact on policy makers and voters, but putting these stories in front of them can be challenging. It can be intimidating for people to share their private lives to wide audiences, and most people rarely have the luxury of time to meet with officials. These comics made it possible for patients from the clinic to advocate for themselves and represent their own stories with decision makers, all the while looking the reader in the eye as they tell of their everyday struggles with health care access.

Comics Collectives: Other Activism Projects

The precursor to the *Sketches Outside the Margins* project was *Comics 4 Health Coverage*, my first foray into organizing cartoonists around a cause. In 2013, the first year that the ACA made health insurance widely available, a group of cartoonists joined me in putting out a call for four panels about why health insurance matters. Our idea was to encourage dialogue on what it means to have (or not have) insurance as way of drawing attention to the availability of coverage, especially for healthier young people upon whom the viability of the ACA depended, and the need to expand the program.

The call resulted in submissions from cartoonists in the local Seattle region as well as a few from across the country and even a couple from outside the country (where some people are mystified by the United States' health care system). We posted the submissions to a Facebook account, which also allowed others to partake in the conversation via the comments. Several of the submissions chronicled the long-term consequences of the lack of coverage. Others, like Kelly Froh's "Lumps," illustrated how access to care can alleviate the anxiety of undiagnosed symptoms.

Another comics activism project developed organically after the 2018 shootings at Stoneman Douglas High School in Parkland, Florida. I was unnerved by a news interview with a teacher who was willing to risk his life to save his students, and I channeled the flood of emotions into a draft of a comic. Working with Mita Mahato as coeditor, we reached out to other cartoonists who are parents and teachers to put together a series of comics. Under the title *Lines Drawn: Parents and Teachers Who've Had Enough*, we expressed our anguish toward gun violence in schools. *MUTHA Magazine*, an edgy online parenting publication, published the comics in two parts, and a selection of the series was also published online on *Illustrated PEN*.

In both the *Comics 4 Health Coverage* and *Lines Drawn* projects, the personal perspectives and internal narratives that can be represented through the comics form lent emotional weight to current public health issues. Whereas the comics journalism of the *Sketches Outside the Margins* project gave voice to the patients interviewed, the voices in these two projects are much more interior. They directly express the cartoonists' fears and anxieties, or sometimes relief and gratitude. Because they are in comics form, we see how the cartoonists experience these emotions, what thoughts flash through their heads, and what triggers their emotional responses. Sometimes the calls to action are literal. In others, the horrible absurdity of the situation—whether it's preschoolers preparing for gun violence or the shocking debt incurred by a medical necessity—implicitly call for change.

Telling the Stories from the Public Health Frontlines

When public health is functioning well—in other words, if people aren't suffering from poor air quality, food-borne illness, infectious disease outbreaks, or other ailments related to conditions in their communities—it's easy for the work that makes that possible to go unnoticed. But with increasing budget cuts across health departments and taxpayers who feel overburdened, we need to tell the stories about what we do and the value we add in ensuring the safety of food and water, the containment of infectious disease, and the prevention of chronic illness in our communities.

Telling the story of a local health department is complicated when there are many interests at play, and garnering support for resourcing a government agency is always a bit of a tough sell. Elected officials and department heads have a vested interest in simultaneously showing how effective the public health system is and demonstrating the constraints of poor funding. It's a delicate balance. The public does not want to pour more money into a system perceived as dysfunctional, and yet the system can't be fully functional without better funding.

Comics offer a communication tool that can add the human elements to this narrative and show the value of public health in a compelling visual style. "Stretched Thin: An Outbreak Story," one of the comics that opens this chapter, is a behind-the-scenes tour of the magnitude of the work of a disease investigation unit. At the same time, the comic touches upon the personal toll a monthslong mumps outbreak response took on this high-performing staff, as personified by disease case reports shrilly demanding their attention. Most importantly, the "Stretched Thin" comic drew attention to how easily a highly competent and skilled public health team could be stretched past capacity if a major outbreak emerged on top of their current workload.

"Stretched Thin" highlighted the work of just one program, but health departments cover a broad range of services that receive little attention despite the value they offer. I had wanted to create comics that tell the many stories of the health department for a few years, but never felt that I had the time to do it. But following Lynda Barry's approach to quickly drawn comics using cheap office supplies, I found that using legal pads and Papermate Flair pens liberated me to quickly sketch snapshots of what the health department does. This has evolved into an occasional web comic strip, *The Public Health Notebook*, that shares accessible public health stories from the health department's social media platforms.

Every day there are fascinating, occasionally horrifying, and frequently moving stories taking place in the public health sector. The proliferation of graphic medicine stories about the experiences of frontline health care staff during the COVID-19 pandemic showed what medical professionals endured during this global crisis; similar stories could be told about public health professionals. As graphic public health develops, I look forward to seeing more of these stories, which can help shine a spotlight on the value of public health programs.

5.

Making Comics for Public Health and Public Information

Perhaps you've been inspired to embark on using comics to communicate about health issues. Or perhaps you are a comics artist who'd like to draw attention to an issue that matters deeply to you. Or maybe you are a communications professional, ready to try developing a comic for public information even though you've never drawn much more than a stick figure.

When I started making public health comics, I was an experienced public health communications professional but I was not well versed in the medium of comics. But I had the benefit of meeting and working alongside talented comics artists who helped me learn as we collaborated. I also live in a city with an active and welcoming comics community, so I had access to workshops, classes, and comics artists who gave me advice and answered my questions. Over the years, I've combined my training in professional health communications with what I've learned about making comics to develop a process for producing graphic public health content. What follows is the advice that I would have given myself as I was starting out writing and making comics for health communication.

A Comics Education

If you are new to comics, start reading more comics. The range of styles, voices, and narrative choices is amazingly broad, and diving in will give you a sense of what's possible. Find some graphic novels at the library or search for web comics online. Look for comics festivals or comic conventions in your area—even the big conventions usually have an artist alley where you can peruse independent comics and meet the artists.

As you read, pay attention to the techniques the authors use. What kind of information can you glean just from the images? How does the dialogue move the story along? How does your eye flow through the comic, and what makes some comics read more easily than others? How do sound effects, visual angle changes, and pacing affect your understanding? Notice which comics stay with you long after you've finished reading and make you think about them afterward, then consider what made them compelling.

If you are in the health field, a good place to start is with the online graphic medicine community found at graphicmedicine.org. They've reviewed and listed an ever-growing number of graphic novels, web comics, and other comics that address health issues as told by patients, health care providers, bioethicists, caregivers, health educators, and other cartoonists. Some of the social commentary comics on sites like *The Nib* (thenib.com), *MUTHA Magazine* (muthamagazine.com), *Illustrated PEN* (pen.org) and the longer-format comics on *The New Yorker* online offer good models for public information comics.

There are also many excellent resource books to help orient you to comics development. Two authors/artists whom I have found helpful and inspiring are Scott McCloud and Lynda Barry. *Understanding Comics* and its companion volume, *Making Comics*, by McCloud artfully explain the mechanics of comics and how they are used to construct meaning. These two books are primers on the comics medium and will hone your appreciation for the nuances and communicative power of comics. Lynda Barry, a legendary cartoonist and teacher, explores writing with images in her books *Making Comics*, *What It Is*, and *Picture This*, with writing and drawing exercises that will stretch your creativity and give you practice as a visual storyteller.

Concept Development: The Creative Brief

Public information comics follow a different development process than comics that are made for mainly artistic or self-expression purposes. As public information, they often require a clearer correspondence between the intended meaning and the meaning received by the reader. Even if you have a strong idea already in mind for a public information comic, grounding your comic in basic health communications practice will compel you to clearly define your purpose in creating the comic—and that will more likely result in a comic that will have the impact you desire.

A creative strategy brief is a common communications tool that can enhance clarity of purpose before you begin writing, drawing, or hiring an artist. For those who are not familiar with this practice, I'll walk you through the steps.

Communication Objectives

First, clarify what you're trying to achieve. Determine what you want to happen as a result of this comic by considering what you want the reader to think, feel, or do after reading it. Are you trying to:

- create awareness of an issue?
- enhance knowledge on a topic?
- make an emotional appeal?
- promote a different way to look at an issue or cultural change?
- promote behavior change or a call to action?

Target Audiences

Identify the audience you are trying to reach with this comic. This could be broad or specific, depending on your communication objectives. It may include multiple audiences. Consider:

- *How will reaching this audience help you meet your communication objectives?* Make sure you identify the right audiences to meet the objectives.
- *What do you know about this audience?* Who do they find credible and trust as sources of information on this topic? What do they care about and what are strongly held values? How do they feel about your organization or affiliation (if applicable)? You may need to find key informants or cultural navigators who can help you answer these questions.
- *What do they know about this issue and how do they feel about it?* What experiences have they had related to this issue? What are possible knowledge gaps? What sensitivities do you need to take into account?

Key Messages

Before you write any part of the comic, flesh out the top messages that the reader should walk away with after reading it. These messages won't necessarily be directly stated in the text of the comic, but readers should arrive at the meaning of the messages through its combination of images, words, dialogue, and sequencing. Formally articulating these messages will help you stay focused in the development process; it's easy to lose the purpose once you get into the creative development if you don't have the key messages as guideposts.

Communication Tactics and Creative Development

Once you have established objectives, articulated key messages, and identified your audiences, you are ready to plan the communication tactics that you'll use.

Are Comics the Right Choice?

Before launching into the creative development, pause to consider whether comics are the appropriate medium for communicating with this audience and these objectives. Most of the time, I think the answer is *yes*, but that may not always be the case. Some audiences might find comics on a given topic off-putting or may not see comics as a credible way to provide information; others may not benefit from the visual nature of this medium. But these audiences are the exception.

A note of caution: if you ask some audiences whether they would like information in comics form, they may not yet have enough familiarity with the possibilities of comics to know whether it will appeal to them. I have found that some groups associate comics so strongly with superheroes or the Sunday funnies that they initially don't think they would like public information comics. But when the same people see a draft of a public health comic, they have often expressed enthusiasm for information presented this way.

Approach, Appeal, and Tone

With your objectives and audience in mind, think about what overall communication approach, look, and feel will be most effective. These decisions will be the most influential in giving shape to your comic.

Your approach to the presentation of information depends on your objectives. Didactic instructional comics may work well to demonstrate a behavior (such as how to prevent germ transmission) or explain how a process occurs (like the buildup of greenhouse gases). A more narrative, storytelling style may be effective when your objective is creating awareness or evoking an emotional response. However, there is no *one* formula for different communication objectives, and much will depend on the topic and the audience. Didactic health education comics can also serve an awareness function and may be necessary when the topic is unfamiliar (such as how to use a medicine return drop box). Storytelling could be used to demonstrate specific behaviors through the course of the story (such as how to be ready for disasters) and may make an otherwise lackluster topic more appealing. Comics journalism—using comics as a form of reporting—is an exciting genre that can be highly informative while keeping a strong narrative.

Closely related are the appeal and tone of the comics. The variety of comics genres is almost dizzying. They include graphic memoir, independent and small press comics, manga, superhero comics, underground comix, art house comics, and plenty of comics that defy genre. Different styles of comics will convey different moods and tones, and some may be more inviting or engaging to your target audience than others. It may be more helpful to think about the general feel you want the comic to have: are you aiming for a comic that is friendly, high energy, calm, edgy, or visually arresting, for instance? Identifying approach, appeal, and tone will set the direction for writing a script and selecting an artist.

Other Early Considerations

Identification of Potential Challenges and Barriers

Early in the development process, try to anticipate any considerations that may require additional planning so that you can reach your objectives. What cultural and language considerations should you address? Are there entrenched views or political sensitivities that you should take into account? Do you have limited resources that you can use to create the comic? Plan ahead so that you can make adjustments.

Distribution

A public information comic won't have an impact if the public never sees it. How will you get the comic in front of your target audience? Determining your distribution method is critical because it dictates many formatting decisions. Some options include:

- *Web*: Where will it be housed online? How will people find it?
- *Social media*: What size and what number of panels will work best for the platform? Can some information be part of the text in the post that accompanies the comic?
- *Print*: How will you distribute printed copies? What budget do you have for printing costs? Can you afford color, heavier paper, cutting, folding, stapling?
- *Outdoor advertising*: If you plan to use the comics as billboards, bus ads, or other outdoor ads, how will you make them easy to read from a distance?

Writing for Public Information Comics

Over time, I have come up with my own processes for writing public information comics informed by my other public health communications work, but you may find a method that works better for you. I share mine as examples to get those new to comics started.

Conversations with Subject Matter Experts

Key messages are always central to the development of any public information. I rarely state the key messages word for word in the comic, but I mull over how the *meanings* in the key messages could come across clearly in the comics form. Often, I'm working with subject matter experts, such as epidemiologists, disease experts, or health educators. They guide me in developing the communication objectives, writing key messages, and identifying the target audiences. Creative ideas often develop as I ask them questions about what is most important for the audience to know and what challenges they've experienced in communicating the topic.

For example, in developing the Don't Hang on to Meds comics campaign, a program manager who works on opioid overdose prevention pointed me to an audio recording. It was of a young woman recounting how her opioid use started when she took pills out of her family's medicine cabinet. This real-life story was utterly compelling, and the young woman telling it was a credible voice for the rationale for medicine return. It prompted me to think about how we could use the auto-bio style of comics to tell similar stories from the perspectives of different people affected by easy access to medications.

Contemplating How the Image Can Carry Meaning

Sometimes it's easier to start by thinking about the images. Are there any images that could be particularly evocative in conveying the meaning of the key messages? Practice "writing" in both words and images. You don't have to be a great artist to do this—stick figures and blobby shapes can work—but you do need to flex your visual creativity.

I started writing my first comic, *No Ordinary Flu*, with a specific image in mind. I wanted to convey how daily life was radically changed during the 1918 influenza pandemic due to illness and infection control measures. I pictured a solitary figure walking past an empty playground after schools were shuttered to prevent the spread of flu. That visual idea served as the spark of a story about a family living through the 1918 pandemic.

Storyboarding helped me solidify my ideas. I was brand-new to writing comics, and I found it helpful to use a pad of paper intended for storyboarding comics, with squares for sketching alongside a space for writing text (fig. 5.1). This type of layout may prompt you to think about both the visuals and text and how they will fit together. I gave a draft of the storyboard to the artist, David Lasky, to help communicate what I envisioned, and also gave him leeway to suggest alternatives to my storyboard panels (fig. 5.2).

For those who are inclined to sketch their visual ideas, storyboards are great tools, and you can do them most efficiently if you do the illustrations as "thumbnails." Thumbnails are small, quick sketches to get the general visual idea or composition roughed out. You can include the text in the thumbnail to help you get an idea of how the text will fit—it's also a reminder to keep the text minimal! Or you can leave out the text and just roughly sketch the images to get an idea of how the images will flow.

COMIC BOOK LAYOUT PAGE
14/15
[Arturo walking on a near empty street.]
Almost overnight, their world changed.
16
[Arturo walks past closed theater.]
CLOSED BY ORDER OF HEALTH DEPA
CLOSED
14
[Arturo walks past empty playground]

SHE'S DELIRIOUS. I'LL TAKE CARE OF HER, ARTURO. FILL IN FOR ME AT THE STORE.
THEATER
CLOSED
SPECIAL

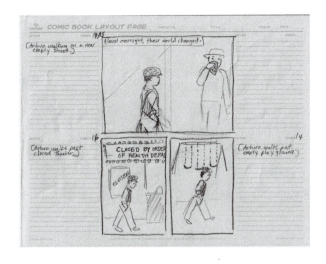

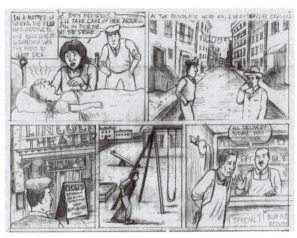

Fig. 5.1. A storyboard roughly sketched out by the author for *No Ordinary Flu.* The storyboard helped convey to the artist what the author envisioned and also helped communicate about the project to others in the health department.

Fig. 5.2. A rough draft of the same page by David Lasky shows how the artist refined the storyboard concept.

Tracking the Elements Through a Script

I often begin writing a script in a table format to get down the basic structure of the story and the flow of written information. Scripts in table form can help track how the elements of a comic will work together during the writing process. Each panel gets a row, with separate columns for the text and the images (table 1). After the first draft, I review it, looking for opportunities to replace the written word with images, sequences or dialogue. I'll often write in this table format before I make the thumbnails, then adjust the script after I have a sense of how this will look visually. Once a pretty solid script draft has come together, I meet with the artist to receive their input on how the images and text will work together. This leads to additional rounds of script revisions before the artist begins to draw a first draft of the comic.

Table 1 Script from lead testing comic

Panel	Text	Image
Cover page	*Why Testing for Lead Helps Kids and Their Growing Brains*	Row of kids, from babies to late elementary school.
Inside cover (1)	Lead is a metal that is poisonous if it gets in your body. Children who are six and younger are the most likely to be harmed by lead. They can get lead poisoning from sources of lead inside the home and outdoors.	Little kids.
2	Even small amounts of lead can harm your child's brain growth. If lead gets into your child, it can make it hard for them to learn, pay attention, and do well in school.	Make the child look younger (3–4 years old). Child on floor raising hand, with a circle outside the child's body showing what the brain looks like, pointing at the child's head.
3	Teacher: "I've been teaching preschool for fifteen years. "I found out that lead poisoning can be a reason why some children have a hard time in school."	
4	Teacher: "But the earlier it's diagnosed, the more we can do to help that child."	Teacher working with child. Make the child look younger (3–4 years old).
5	Kids get lead poisoning from swallowing lead. Lead is in dust and chips from paint in older homes. Paint dust is one of the main sources of lead poisoning.	Inside older home, parent nailing a picture on a wall with a shelf of toys underneath. Dust falls from the nailing activity.

Finding the Right Artist

A Word for Amateur Cartoonists, or Those Who Would Like to Give It a Try

The first consideration related to working with an artist is: could it be you? The answer may be an obvious yes or no as you read this. But if you are at all visually inclined and the idea of drawing comics yourself is intriguing, there are ways to develop your skill so that you could do the artwork, depending on the objectives of your comic.

I enjoyed drawing as a teen and had some minimal drawing instruction in high school, after which I largely stopped drawing for over twenty years. After working with David Lasky on *No Ordinary Flu*, I took one of his workshops on making auto-bio comics. Lasky always makes a point to tell his students that you don't have to be a top-notch artist to create good comics, but you do need to be a good storyteller. He pointed out a number of legendary cartoonists, like Charles Schultz and Matt Groening, who were not the best technical artists but drew with expression, wrote stories that connected, and were masters of the comic form. That class gave me the courage to start making my own comics. My confidence was further bolstered by attending the international Comics & Medicine conferences, where all attendees were encouraged to sketch and share their work as part of the graphic medicine community. I enrolled in workshops from Short Run Comix and Arts, a nonprofit organization in Seattle, and through this organization, I met other cartoonists who encouraged me—and from whom I continue to learn.

It has taken some years, but I am much more confident in calling myself a cartoonist and I now create comics both as a writer and artist. If you want to try cartooning, you may be able to build up your skills by looking for classes in making comics at art schools, art centers, community colleges, and recreational programs. The practice of making comics and sharing them with other comics makers—and asking questions about how they make comics—has also been instrumental in helping me improve. There are many comics artists on social media, which can be a great way to interact with those with more experience and to see how others tell their stories. My cartooning is still a work in progress!

In my day job at a public health department, I still mainly hire and collaborate with professional artists. I lack time to do the artwork, and I also hire professionals who can often deliver the right look and feel for a particular audience. My own comics are well suited to relatively quick stories for the health department's blog or for my personal public health activism. But for larger campaigns or comics that will get greater exposure, professional and more experienced comics artists can provide a more polished result.

Where to Find Comics Artists

I was lucky the first time I sought a comics artist. I had no background in comics, but I live in a city with a thriving comics community, and I knew someone-who-knew-someone in the comics world. But not everyone may be able to find artists by word of mouth. Fortunately, there are other strategies that may work to help identify comics talent-for-hire.

- *Follow Graphic Medicine.* There is an international community, including many artists, with a shared interest in the intersection of comics and health. Following the Graphic Medicine social media feeds (@graphicmedicine) and blog (graphic-medicine.org) will help you identify potential artists.
- *Scout local comics festivals.* Search online for comics festivals or comics conventions in your area. Festivals that feature independent comics, small press comics, and zines are promising places to actually talk to the artists about their work; you may also find a wide variety of styles among the artists. Examples of independent comics festivals include Small Press Expo (SPX) in Bethesda, Maryland; Chicago Alternative Comics Expo (CAKE); Comic Arts Brooklyn (CAB); Vancouver Comics

Arts Festival (VanCAF); Cartoon Crossroads Columbus (CXC); Massachusetts Independent Comics Expo (MICE); Comics Arts Los Angeles (CALA); and Short Run Comix and Arts Festival in Seattle. Even large comic conventions often have "artist alleys" where the artists are there in person. Note that at the big comic conventions there may be fewer artists who do freelance work or noncommercial work, and some may work at a higher pay scale.

- *Search social media and online.* Many cartoonists have websites or social media presences. If you come across graphic novels, web comics, or other comics that interest you, look for the cartoonist on social media. Following one artist will usually lead to suggestions for other artists to follow. Some of these artists may do freelance work. You can also do online searches for cartoonists in your area.

- *Work with students.* Many art schools, art centers, community colleges, and recreation programs have classes in making comics. You might be able to find a rising comics artist looking for opportunities to work in the medium. A note of caution: some students of comics may produce good-looking work but may not be skilled in storytelling or may be unfamiliar with professional working processes. Some art students may produce gorgeous artwork but not know how to work in the comics medium. Be prepared to be an art director as well as a writer in the process.

- *Use communications and graphic design agencies.* These agencies often work with pools of illustrators, and some illustrators can make quality comics. As with students, these illustrators may not be familiar with how to work in comics, so you should be prepared to be an art director and writer. This can also be a more expensive alternative because the agency will add an overhead charge. You can also work directly with illustrators, but make sure you get a sense of whether they can work well in comics. For example, do they do illustrations that support a narrative or storytelling?

Selecting a Comics Artist

When selecting an artist for a project, consider several factors to find the right fit:

- Does the artist have experience working on commissions? Those who have this experience will know to expect specific deadlines and deliverables. Artists who are new to the process of working with a client may still do a fine job but may require more attention and communication.

- Is the artist's style a good fit for the project? For instance, if you are doing a comic that needs to show people, make sure that the artist is skilled at drawing people. Will the style convey the tone you want to create (such as a lighthearted style to attract parents of young children or an edgy style to appeal to teens and young adults)? Ask to see a portfolio of work to see the artist's different styles.

- Meet with the artist to find out how well the artist communicates, listens, and understands what your objectives are. You may find that the artist has a passion for the topic, and that will likely make for an even better comic. If the artist appears to have little interest in the topic, it may be better to keep looking for the right fit.

Develop a Scope of Work

Create a scope of work for the project that sets clear expectations about what your role will be and what is expected of the artist. This should be done in consultation with the artist, who may have a better understanding of what options are available and what is feasible in the time frame and budget.

A scope of work may include:

- *A description of the project*: Provide a clear understanding of the objectives, the target audiences, and how the comic will be used and distributed.
- *An outline of roles*: This can include delineation of who will develop the key messages and the script, how vetting and approval will happen, how the artist will get access to reference photos or background materials, what role the artist will have in providing input on the script, and what role you (or others) will have in providing input on the artwork.
- *A timeline and/or key milestones*: When will you provide materials to the artist (e.g., scripts, reference materials)? How many rounds of review will this involve? How quickly will feedback and approvals be given to the artist? How quickly will the artist need to provide revisions?
- *Payment instructions*: How much will the artist be paid and who should be invoiced? How will costs incurred (such as printing) be handled? What additional costs may be incurred due to unforeseen revisions?
- *The expected deliverables*: Specify the format you expect to receive. Will the artist handle the printing, or will you? Who will retain the original artwork? Will you receive electronic files, and if so, what type of files?

Collaborating with Comics Artists

I prefer collaborations with comics artists to working entirely on my own. I find that the collaborative process results in better ideas and creative concepts. Having more than one perspective on how to tell the story or convey health information results in a stronger final piece. A successful collaboration depends on having a good working process and clear understanding of what roles each of you will play.

Compensate the Artist

If you are reading this book, you likely know that public health agencies and organizations usually work in resource-strapped environments. However, even in the context of public health, artists need to be compensated for their skill and time. Too often they are asked to work for reduced wages or even for free. Plan for compensation when pursuing grants or developing budgets. Look for grants that fund this type of innovative health communication. Plan to pay a comics artist in the same range you would pay a graphic designer or illustrator.

Roles in the Process

In addition to artwork creation, there are additional roles and responsibilities that you can delegate to the hired artist, or you can choose to take them on yourself. These include:

- *Approach and script development*: A comics artist could develop the approach and the script using the key messages. In this case, the subject matter expert should provide feedback to ensure that the key messages are still intact and that the script aligns with the communications objectives. This works best if the comics artist has experience working for clients or has work in their portfolio that demonstrates the ability to clearly convey information or distinct messages. Rather than leaving it to a comics artist, you could also develop the approach and the script. In this case, involve the artist with your ideas and review of the script. The artist may have good insights for how comics can most effectively be used to relay the messages and may be able to spot potential pitfalls, so it's important to discuss both the approach and script together. In other words, collaboration is essential, no matter who does the writing.
- *Art direction*: You can play a central role in art direction or a much smaller role, but you will need to provide the artist with some level of feedback on the look of the comic as it develops. Art direction can include instructions about character development or the overall aesthetic and tone. You may want to incorporate suggestions for the visuals within the script, but I recommend staying open to ideas that the artist may have. I've found that many times artists have had clearer or more creative ways to represent the script.

And you could rely on the artist heavily for the visual elements. However, even if the artist makes most of the visual decisions, you will need to review early drafts of the artwork. Keep an eye out for any inaccuracies (especially for technical aspects, such as making sure that the depiction of health issues is accurate), make sure that you can follow the logical flow of the panels, and consider whether the comic has the needed feel and tone.

Examples of Visual Choices and Collaboration

Character Development

For the children's emergency preparedness comic book *Ready Freddie!*, I wanted a comic book that wouldn't feel too wholesome in the off-putting way that some educational materials can feel to kids. Artist Thomas Webb proposed two wacky monster children who would be enthusiastic to the point of near mania. My main art direction was to make the characters appear as if they've just eaten too much candy. With that bit of insight, Webb was able to imbue the characters with a zaniness that added just the right irreverence and humor (fig. 5.3).

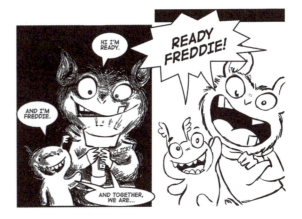

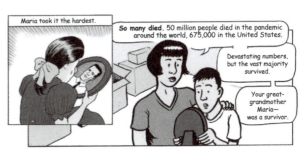

Line Work and Detail

When I worked with David Lasky on *No Ordinary Flu*, we aimed to create images of the 1918 influenza pandemic that have the feel of photographs of that era. Lasky used detailed, finely lined drawings reminiscent of turn-of-the-century publications. He also made the key suggestion to draw the part of the story set in the current day in a modern, clean-lined style (fig. 5.4). His visual device helps the reader understand the different parts of the narrative in a simple way.

HI I'M READY.
AND I'M FREDDIE.
CLICK!
AND TOGETHER, WE ARE...
READY FREDDIE!

Maria took it the hardest.
So many died. 50 million people died in the pandemic around the world, 675,000 in the United States.
Devastating numbers, but the vast majority survived.
Your great-grandmother Maria— was a survivor.

Fig. 5.3. For emergency preparedness comic books aimed at children, we designed monster characters that we hoped would avoid the saccharine, overly wholesome feel of some children's educational materials. The monsters' irreverent personalities were based on children who have eaten too much candy. Artwork by Thomas Webb. Courtesy of Public Health—Seattle & King County.

Fig. 5.4. The shift in narrative between a story about people enduring the 1918 flu pandemic and the story of their descendants is marked by a change from the detailed linework in the first panel to the smoother, thicker lines in the second panel. Artwork by David Lasky for *No Ordinary Flu*. Courtesy of Public Health—Seattle & King County.

Emotional Tone

The emotional tone of the comics deserves particular attention to make sure it's appropriate for how readers already feel about an issue. The emotional tone should also align with the desired impact on the reader: will it help them reach the desired health decision? This is particularly important for comics dealing with issues that can produce high anxiety.

In comics for use in emergency response situations, the facial expressions on the emergency responders are concerned but calm and confident, intended to influence how the public feels about those who are making emergency response decisions. Similarly, when depicting characters in the midst of disasters or outbreaks, it doesn't feel authentic to show them smiling. But even when they are shown as alarmed or distressed, the characters still model an ability to function and make necessary decisions—a quality we want to encourage in the public during disasters.

Palette

The color choices in a comic influence its emotional tone and appeal. When a comic deals with an issue that some people shy away from, colors may make it more inviting. For example, in *Why Testing for Lead Helps Kids and Their Growing Brains*, Amy Camber's use of soft pastels with black and white make a tough subject more approachable; the palette also signals that the subject matter is about young children and babies (see fig. 3.2).

The Don't Hang on to Meds comics campaign promoted medicine return as a way to prevent addiction and suicide. We didn't want to dwell on the darkness of the topic; instead, the focus was on the benefits of actions that prevent the misuse of medications. Artist Tatiana Gill chose vivid, sunny colors that projected optimism and positivity. The palette also made a more effective campaign in drawing the eye to the images as they were shown on the sides of buses, on social media, and in transit terminals (see fig. 3.1).

In 2018, David Lasky and I created *Pandemic in Seattle*, a serialized web comic to commemorate the centennial of the 1918 influenza pandemic (and the tenth anniversary of our first comic, *No Ordinary Flu*). To connect the comic to 1918, Lasky created a palette that evoked the color of newspaper comics in the early twentieth century (see the panels in chapter 2).

Comics in Translation

Comics can be an effective communication medium in translation, as discussed in chapter 2. Compared to other print materials, comics usually have a lower word count, which makes them cheaper to translate than other written materials.

However, translated text presents some unique challenges for comics. In addition to finding quality translators, you will need to plan for inserting translated text into the comics. I recommend using InDesign, Photoshop, Procreate, or another software program that allows you to put the text in a layer separate from the images. That way you can replace the English text with the other language(s).

Table 2 Script translation matrix

Panel	English text	Somali text	Notes to translator
Cover page	*Why Testing for Lead Helps Kids and Their Growing Brains*	*Sababta Baaritaanka macdanta Leedhka u kaalmeeyo Ilmaha iyo Maskaxkooda Koraysa*	
Inside cover (1)	Lead is a metal that is poisonous if it gets in your body. Children who are six and younger are the most likely to be harmed by lead. They can get lead poisoning from sources of lead inside the home and outdoors.	Leedhka waa macdan sun ah haddii ay gasho jirkaaga. Carruurta lix jir ka ah ama ka yar waxay u badan tahay in waxyeelo kasoo gaarto macdanta leedhka. [Ilmaha] waxay ku sumoobi karaan sunta macdanta Leedhka. Meelaha sunta kasoo gaadhana waxay noqon karaan guriga gudahiisa iyo dibaddisa.	
2	Even small amounts of lead can harm your child's brain growth. If lead gets into your child, it can make it hard for them to learn, pay attention, and do well in school.	Xitaa wax yar oo macdanta leedhka ah waxay wax yeelleyn kartaa koritaanka maskaxda ilmahaaga. Haddii uu leedhka ilmahaaga saameeyo, waxay ku adkeyn kartaa in ay wax bartaan, feejignaadaan, iyo in ay ku fiicnaadaan iskuulka.	"gets into": translated as affects.

When the artist designs the placement of text, leave extra space for translated text. Some languages, like Russian or Spanish, use more words or have longer words. Other languages, like Chinese or Korean, tend to take up less space. And a few languages, like Arabic, read right to left, with book pages running in the opposite direction, requiring the images to flip in order for speech or thought bubbles to read correctly.

If the artist does not read the language, you will also need to plan for how to put the correct translated text in the right spot. If you use the table format shown in table 2, you can put each English sentence in a row with a column next to it for a translator to insert the corresponding translated text. That way, you'll know what the translation says so that you can identify where it goes in the comic.

Another consideration is the font type in translation. If you want the lettering to look similar in multiple languages, use a common TrueType font such as Arial, Times, or (gasp!) even Comic Sans. TrueType fonts work for most languages.

Testing, Vetting, and Evaluation

One of my favorite things about working in comics is the iterative process of talking through ideas with artists and then seeing the big reveal of their first draft. When I get a new draft—after I'm past the initial giddiness of seeing the artwork realized—I do a careful review to make sure that the key messages are clear and the informational objectives of the comic are met. Often this also involves a round of review from subject matter experts who helped develop the key messages. You may need to tweak the text once you see how it's working (or not working) with the images and suggest adjustments to the images for clarity, emotional tone, and appeal to target audiences.

It's best if you have the opportunity to do formative testing of drafts of the comics with members of the target audience before the final inking is done. For example, we tested comics about norovirus and flu prevention using intercept surveys with patients in the waiting room of public health clinics. For a mini-comic about lead poisoning, environmental health staff brought draft copies of a comic book to meetings with immigrant community members for their review; these community members provided feedback about both the content of the comic books and the translation. It's easier to recruit reviewers if you provide some kind of compensation, such as grocery store gift cards, and it's also an appropriate way to demonstrate the value placed on their time and expertise. We've also recruited reviewers from community organizations that are already partners in public health projects. Feedback from the intended audiences helps refine the text and the illustrations for clarity and cultural relevance.

Questions for formative review could include:

- If you saw this comic book sitting in a waiting room, would you pick it up? Why or why not?
- What were the main ideas you learned from reading this?
- Was there anything in this comic strip that was confusing?
- Was there anything in this comic strip that didn't reflect your community or was offensive in your culture?
- Would other people you know read information presented in this way? Why or why not?
- How was the quality of the translation?

Evaluation of the effectiveness of comics to reach their intended objectives is a final important part of the process of health communications. Unfortunately, like for many other forms of health communication, evaluation often is not prioritized in funding for comics projects; as other health communication efforts demand attention in a resource-strapped environment, evaluation is often overlooked. Much of the feedback I've received on the comics work has been anecdotal rather than formal evaluation, typically in form of responses from community partners who express appreciation for providing communication that speaks to their constituents.

However, evaluation that would provide more understanding of this medium in health communication would consider these questions:

- How well do comics draw people's attention?
- Do comics appeal to people in target audiences? Why or why not?
- As a result of reading a public health comic, how much awareness do people have about a health issue? How well do they remember the key messages presented? Did reading the comic affect their attitudes or knowledge about a health issue? How likely are they to perform health behaviors promoted in a public health comic?
- How credible are comics as a source of health information?
- What uses of comics reach people from target audiences best (e.g., online, billboards, bus ads, comic books, etc.)?
- How do audiences engage with the information when presented as comics?

What Makes the Best Graphic Public Health

I hope that sharing what I've learned in graphic public health projects will encourage others to tell stories and make comics about public health—or about the environment, education, transportation, or whatever public issue ignites their passion. More than any technique or method for making comics, calling upon that passion makes good public information comics. If you can tap into *why* you care about what you're messaging, and you remain focused on the end goal of changing behaviors, hearts, and minds, it will show in the themes, writing, and images in your comic.

The field of public health is packed with gripping, occasionally funny, and often emotional stories about dedicated public health workers, resilient people, vibrant communities, and issues that deeply matter. During the COVID-19 pandemic, amazing, inspiring comics proliferated about the experiences of people during this massive public health emergency.[1] But it doesn't take a pandemic to tell a compelling graphic health story; comics could powerfully tell why the health of people in some neighborhoods is so much better than the health of people just miles away, or what happens in the typical day of a restaurant inspector, or what happened on the front lines of the Ebola response in West Africa, or how vaping products infiltrated American schools. Graphic public health offers a creatively fertile medium with the potential to connect public health to human faces, facilitate understanding of actionable health information, and illuminate public health's key role within people's lives and in their communities.

There are so many good graphic public health stories waiting. I can't wait to read them all.

Notes

Chapter 1

1. McCloud, *Understanding Comics*, 60–93.
2. Chute, *Why Comics?*, 23.
3. Gazmarian et al., "Public Health Literacy in America," 319–20.
4. Freeman et al., "Public Health Literacy Defined," 447–48.
5. See Taylor's work for *The Nib*, including "Black Mothers Face Far Worse Outcomes" and "America Isn't Ready for a Pandemic"; Gharib's work for NPR's *Goats and Soda*, including "A Day in Coronavirus Awareness Mode" and "How to Fight Menstrual Stigma"; and Neufeld's "A Tale of Two Pandemics."
6. McNichol, "Potential of Educational Comics," 27.
7. Chute and Jagoda, "Comics and Media," 4.
8. Chute, *Why Comics?*, 22.
9. Cited in conversation in ibid., 23–24.
10. For more on interactive health literacy, see Nutbeam, "Health Literacy."
11. Ibid.; Sykes et al., "Understanding Critical Health Literacy."
12. McNichol, "Potential of Educational Comics."

Chapter 2

1. Chute, *Why Comics?*, 34.

Chapter 3

1. CDC, 4-H, and USDA, *Junior Disease Detectives*.

Chapter 4

1. Pigg, "Things Anthropologists Can Do."
2. Ibid.

Chapter 5

1. See Boileau and Johnson, *COVID Chronicles*, and COVID-19 comics in Bors, "Pandemic Issue" of *The Nib*, and referenced in Aguiar, "Through Comics."

Bibliography

Aguiar, Annie. "Through Comics, Seattle Cartoonists Document Their Lives During the Coronavirus Pandemic." *Seattle Times*, June 12, 2020. https://www.seattletimes .com/entertainment/visual-arts/seattle -cartoonists-document-their-lives-in-these -coronavirus-times-through-comics.

Andreasen, Alan R. "Social Marketing: Definition and Domain." *Journal of Public Policy and Marketing* 13, no. 1 (1994): 108–14.

Boileau, Kendra, and Rich Johnson. *COVID Chronicles: A Comics Anthology*. University Park: Graphic Mundi, 2021.

Bors, Matt, ed. "Pandemic Issue." *The Nib* 2, no. 3 (2020).

Centers for Disease Control and Prevention, 4-H, and U.S. Department of Agriculture. *Junior Disease Detectives*. Accessed February 19, 2020. https://www.cdc.gov /flu/resource-center/freeresources/graphic -novel/junior-detectives-print-web.pdf.

Chute, Hillary. *Why Comics: From Underground to Everywhere*. New York: Harper, 2017.

Chute, Hillary, and Patrick Jagoda. "Introduction to Special Issue: Comics and Media." *Critical Inquiry* 40, no. 3 (2014): 1–10.

Freeman, Darcy A., et al. "Public Health Literacy Defined." *American Journal of Preventive Medicine* 36, no. 5 (2009): 446–51.

Gazmararian, Julie A., et al. "Public Health Literacy in America: An Ethical Imperative." *American Journal of Preventive Medicine* 28, no. 3 (2004): 317–22.

Gharib, Malaka. "I Spent a Day in Coronavirus Awareness Mode. Epidemiologists, How Did I Do?" *NPR: Goats and Soda*, March 12, 2020. Accessed April 3, 2021. https:// www.npr.org/sections/goatsand soda/2020/03/12/814414450/comic-i -spent-a-day-in-coronavirus-awareness -mode-epidemiologists-how-did-i-do.

———. "Tips on How to Fight Menstrual Stigma." *NPR: Goats and Soda*, February 19, 2021. Accessed April 3, 2021. https:// www.npr.org/sections/goatsandsoda/2021 /02/19/968404983/why-is-a-red-stain-a -disaster-tips-on-fighting-period-stigma -plus-a-zine.

McCloud, Scott. *Understanding Comics: The Invisible Art*. Northampton, MA: Kitchen Sink Press, 1993.

McNicol, Sarah. "The Potential of Educational Comics as a Health Information Medium." *Health Information and Libraries Journal* 34, no. 1 (2016): 20–31.

Neufeld, Josh. "A Tale of Two Pandemics: A Nonfiction Comic About Historical Racial Health Disparities." *Journalists Resource*, November 16, 2020. Accessed April 3, 2021. https://journalistsresource.org/race-and -gender/pandemics-comic-racial-health -disparities.

Nutbeam, Don. "Health Literacy as a Public Health Goal: A Challenge for Contemporary Health Education and Communication Strategies into the 21st Century." *Health Promotion International* 15, no. 3 (2000): 259–67.

Pigg, Stacy. "Things Anthropologists Can Do with Comics." *Medical Anthropology Quarterly*. March 19, 2018. Accessed July 5, 2021. https://medanthroquarterly.org/ forums/forumreview/things-anthro pologists-can-do-with-comics.

Sykes, Susie, Jane Wills, Gillian Rowlands, and Keith Popple. "Understanding Critical Health Literacy: A Concept Analysis." *Biomed Central Public Health* 13 (2013): 150.

Taylor, Whit. "America Isn't Ready for a Pandemic." *The Nib*, January 8, 2018. Accessed April 3, 2021. https://thenib.com /america-ready-pandemic.

———. "Black Mothers Face Far Worse Health Outcomes. How Do We Fix It?" *The Nib*, February 24, 2020. Accessed April 3, 2021. https://thenib.com/pregnancy-and-race.